OXFORD MEDICAL PUBLICATIONS

Psychopharmacology of
Panic

BRITISH ASSOCIATION
FOR PSYCHOPHARMACOLOGY MONOGRAPHS

Psychopharmacology of Panic

BRITISH ASSOCIATION FOR
PSYCHOPHARMACOLOGY MONOGRAPH
No. 12

Edited by

STUART A. MONTGOMERY

Reader and Honorary Consultant
Academic Department of Psychiatry
St Mary's Hospital Medical School

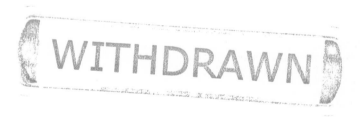

Oxford   New York   Tokyo
OXFORD UNIVERSITY PRESS
1993

Oxford University Press, Walton Street, Oxford OX2 6DP

Oxford New York Toronto
Delhi Bombay Calcutta Madras Karachi
Kuala Lumpur Singapore Hong Kong Tokyo
Nairobi Dar es Salaam Cape Town
Melbourne Auckland Madrid
and associated companies in
Berlin Ibadan

Oxford is a trade mark of Oxford University Press

Published in the United States
by Oxford University Press Inc., New York

A catalogue record for this book is available from the British Library

Library of Congress Cataloging in Publication Data
Psychopharmacology of panic / edited by Stuart A. Montgomery, — 1st
    ed.
    (British Association for Psychopharmacology monograph; no. 12)
    (Oxford medical publications)
    Includes bibliographical references and index.
    1. Panic disorders.   2. Panic disorders—Molecular aspects.
3. Panic disorders—Chemotherapy.   4. Psychopharmacology.
I. Montgomery, S. A.   II. Series.   III. Series: Oxford medical
publications.
    [DNLM: 1. Panic—drug effects.   2. Panic Disorder—drug therapy.
3. Panic Disorder—epidemiology.   4. Psychopharmacology.   W1 BR343D
no. 12 / WM 178 P9735]
RC535.P78   1993   616.85'223—dc20   92–16486

ISBN 0–19–262087–8

Typeset by Graphicraft Typesetters Ltd., Hong Kong
Printed in Great Britain on acid-free paper by
Bookcraft Ltd., Midsomer Norton, Avon

Preface

Panic disorder, now recognized in both the DSM-III, DSM-IV, and ICD-10 diagnostic systems as an important condition, occurs in some 1.5 per cent of the general population and is associated with substantial morbidity. The distress caused by the disorder is reflected in the high rate of attendance at clinics and emergency departments and in the raised suicide rate that is associated with the illness.

The boundaries of the disorder are not yet clearly defined and the evidence of substantial co-morbidity with social phobia has led to the debate about whether or not some of the phobias are secondary to panic disorder. The co-morbidity with depression, particularly recurrent brief depression, creates particular problems in interpreting studies since the evidence suggests that panic disorder with depression has a different pharmacology, and presumably a different underlying biological basis, to pure panic disorder. This has encouraged the study of the condition in the pure form without concomitant depression.

Recent studies have led to the realization that the underlying biochemical and pathophysiological mechanisms are more complex than was originally thought. The more simplistic theories of aetiology that explained panic symptoms in terms of learned misbehaviours have had to be modified or replaced to accommodate findings that point to the importance of the homeostasis of acid–base mechanisms, the finding that CCK-4 may provoke panic, and findings on the importance of serotonergic mechanisms which suggest a more specific biochemical abnormality.

Until recently little guidance could be given about management and treatment. However, panic disorder appears to respond well to treatment and, as the chapters in the book make clear, there is now an increasing body of carefully collected data that will help lead to more informed choices for treatment strategies.

This book provides a collection of critical papers by leading authorities on the subject stemming from an international symposium on panic disorder arranged by the British Association of Psychopharmacology. It brings together in one volume a timely update on the epidemiology and co-morbidity of panic disorders, as well as offering insight into the various theories of the genesis of the disorder, both biochemical and behavioural, and offers advice about various treatment strategies.

London　　　　　　　　　　　　　　　　　　　　　　　　S.A.M.
July 1992

Contents

Contributors

JULES ANGST, *Psychiatric University Hospital Zurich, Research Department, PO Box 68, CH-8029 Zurich, Switzerland.*

G.W. ASHCROFT, *Clinical Trials Unit, Clinical Research Centre, Royal Cornhill Hospital, Cornhill Road, Aberdeen AB922H, UK.*

DAVID BALL, *Reckitt and Colman Psychopharmacology Unit, School of Medical Sciences, University Walk, Bristol BS8 ITD, UK.*

MICHEL BOURIN, *Faculty of Medicine, University of Nantes, 44035 Nantes, France.*

JACQUES BRADWEJN, *McGill University and St Mary's Hospital Centre, 3830 Lacombe Avenue, Montreal, Canada.*

ANDREW C. BRIGGS, *Department of Psychiatry, Clinical Sciences Building, Leicester Royal Infirmary, PO Box 65, Leicester LE2 7LX, UK.*

J. BUTLER, *Pharmacology Department, University College, Galway, Ireland.*

BERNARD J. CARROLL, *Department of Psychiatry, Duke University Medical Center, Box 3414, Durham, NC 27710, USA.*

G.B. CASSANO, *Institute of Clinical Psychiatry, University of Pisa via Roma, 67–56100 Pisa, Italy.*

HANS A. DEN BOER, *Department of Biological Psychiatry, University Hospital Utrecht, PO Box 85500, 3508 GA Utrecht, The Netherlands.*

T.J. FAHY, *Psychiatric Unit, University College Hospital, Galway, Ireland.*

PAUL GLUE, *Reckitt and Colman Psychopharmacology Unit, School of Medical Sciences, University Walk, Bristol BS8 ITD, UK.*

DONALD F. KLEIN, *Department of Psychiatry, College of Physicians and Surgeons of Columbia University, 722 West 168th Street, New York, NY 10032, USA.*

DIANA KOSZYCKI, *St Mary's Hospital Centre, 3830 Lacombe Avenue, Montreal, Canada.*

CHRIS LAWSON, *Reckitt and Colman Psychopharmacology Unit, School of Medical Sciences, University Walk, Bristol BS8 ITD, UK.*

BRIAN E. LEONARD, *Pharmacology Department, University College, Galway, Ireland.*

A. LYLE, *Department of Mental Health, Aberdeen University, Medical School, Foresterhill, Aberdeen AB9 2ZD, UK.*

STUART A. MONTGOMERY, *Academic Department of Psychiatry, St Mary's Hospital Medical School, Praed Street, London W2 1 NY, UK.*

DAVID J. NUTT, *Reckitt and Colman Psychopharmacology Unit, Schoot of Medical Sciences, University Walk, Bristol BS8 ITD, UK.*

D. O'ROURKE, *Psychiatric Unit, University College Hospital, Galway, Ireland.*

RICHARD PAYEUR, *McGill University, St Mary's Hospital Centre, 3830 Lacombe Avenue, Montreal, Canada.*

M. SAVINO, *Institute of Clinical Psychiatry, University of Pisa via Roma, 67–56100, Pisa, Italy.*

R. FIONA STIRTON, *Department of Psychiatry, Clinical Sciences Building, Leicester Royal Infirmary, PO Box 65, Leicester LE2 7LX, UK.*

L.G. WALKER, *Department of Mental Health, Aberdeen University, Medical School, Foresterhill, Aberdeen AB9 2ZD, UK.*

HERMAN G.M. WESTENBERG, *Department of Biological Psychiatry, University Hospital Utrecht, PO Box 85500, 3508 GA, Utrecht, The Netherlands.*

WERNER WICKI, *Psychiatric University Hospital Zurich, Research Department, PO Box 68, CH-8029, Zurich, Switzerland.*

SUE WILSON, *Reckitt and Colman Psychoparmacology Unit, School of Medical Sciences, University Walk, Bristol BS8 ITD, UK.*

1

The areas of clinical and biological advance in panic disorder: an introduction

STUART A. MONTGOMERY

The phenomenon of panic, of extreme fear accompanied by physical symptoms, has had numerous descriptions and different names in the psychiatric literature, but the concept of panic disorder is relatively new in the classifications of psychiatric disorders. The pioneering work of Donald Klein and his associates has drawn attention to the importance of the phenomenon of panic in separating out a group of patients who have a different course of illness, and a different psychopharmacology from other anxiety states (Klein 1964).

Panic disorder was first accepted as a separate diagnostic entity in the Unites States with its inclusion in the DSM-III classification of the American Psychiatric Association in 1980. Some problems of definition still remain however. There is considerable variability in the symptoms, and in the severity and frequency of attacks (Aronson 1987). In DSM-III-R there is some recognition of the difficulty of definition in the, to some extent conflicting, requirements of either four episodes in four weeks or continuous fear of an attack for four weeks.

The definition of panic disorder has changed somewhat over the last decade and has tended to focus on the frequency of panic attacks and the effect of secondary agoraphobia. The question has been raised as to whether the presence of agoraphobia secondary to the anticipatory fear of panic, should alter the minimum number of panic attacks in a given time required in the diagnostic criteria. General agreement on the answers to these questions has not yet been reached, and it is probable that as results from large studies, both short and long term, are completed in panic disorder, data will become available to help clarify the issues.

THE FREQUENCY OF PANIC ATTACKS

The DSM-III-R diagnostic classification categorizes panic disorder with criteria of psychopathology and of frequency. Epidemiological studies provide data which suggest that individuals with less frequent panic attacks may form a different diagnostic subgroup to those with more frequent attacks. These less frequent panickers are currently excluded from the diagnosis of panic disorder in DSM-III-R which focuses entirely on the group with more frequent panic. The rationale for this separation has not been properly examined, nor for that matter are there sufficient studies, either of psychopathology or response to treatment, to help determine whether the less frequent subgroup should be excluded or not. They form a substantial group as the epidemiological surveys have shown with prevalence rates of up to 10 per cent reported for subjects having the same symptoms as required by DSM-III-R but with lower frequency of attacks (von Korff *et al.* 1985).

CO-MORBIDITY OF PANIC DISORDER

Those who suffer from panic disorder have a relatively high attendance rate for treatment, though they do not always seek treatment for the panic alone (Vollrath *et al.* 1990). The constellation of symptoms making up a panic attack is quite easily recognized by patients. Many patients with severe attacks have a feeling of impending doom prior to the attack which they recognize as illness related. Both patients and physicians find it relatively easy to recognize the phenomenon of a panic attack and it would simplify the management of different kinds of psychiatric illness if the importance of panic attacks were recognized.

One issue which is not properly disentangled is the substantial overlap of panic with other disorders, particularly depression. This co-morbidity with depression might be thought to argue against the recognition of panic as a separate disorder. Different studies have reported from 50 to 75 per cent of patients with panic disorder also suffer from major depression (Coryell *et al.* 1988; Stein and Uhde 1986).

In the longitudinal data from the Zurich epidemiological study more than 60 per cent of those with panic suffered from depression in the same year, the commonest association being with recurrent brief depression, followed by major depression (Vollrath and Angst 1989). There is also an association with dysthymia which itself might be accounted for by the overlap with recurrent brief depression. On the other hand the overlap with anxiety disorders, for example, simple phobia, and generalized anxiety disorder, is surprisingly low. In panic without associated depression there is only a weak association with agoraphobia but this association is markedly elevated when panic disorder overlaps with major depression. This suggests that the agoraphobia seen with panic disorder has its closest association with depression, and that the panic agoraphobia complex should be considered separately from the anxiety disorders.

PANIC AND SUICIDAL BEHAVIOUR

There have been a number of reports of a higher than expected risk of suicide with panic disorder (Markowitz *et al.* 1989; Vollrath and Angst 1989). This might be thought to be explained, not as a direct association of panic disorder but rather as a function of co-morbidity. Major depression, for example, carries an increased risk of suicide, and there is a significant overlap between the disorders.

The NIMH Epidemiological Catchment Area (ECA) study controlled for the effect of major depression, however, and still found a high rate of suicide attempts (Johnson *et al.* 1990). In the Zurich study a similar effect was seen with a higher rate of suicide attempts in the group with panic disorder and depression than in either the major depression or the recurrent brief depression group alone (Vollrath and Angst 1989). The increased suicide risk is not seen in those with pure panic disorder without associated depression and it appears that the coexistence of diagnoses signals a more severe group with greater morbidity.

Clearly further studies are needed to elucidate the relationship between panic disorder and depressive states, but the suggestion at the moment is that all studies on panic disorder should document the presence and the severity of concomitant major depression and of recurrent brief depression.

PHARMACOLOGICAL PROVOCATION OF PANIC

One approach in the attempt to elucidate the mechanisms underlying panic disorder has been the use of agents to provoke panic attacks. If certain biochemical manoeuvres are associated with the provocation of panic attacks this might provide the key to finding treatments that would block the attacks. Pharmacological investigation of panic disorder has benefited from the relative ease with which the individual panic attack is recognized and defined. A number of models have been adopted including the use of sodium lactate, of carbon dioxide and cholecystokinin (CCK) as panic provocation agents (Gorman *et al.* 1984; Margraf *et al.* 1986; Bradwejn *et al.* 1991).

The findings with lactate infusions have been quite consistent and appear to differentiate between panic disorder patients and controls (Margraf *et al.* 1986). However, further studies suggest that the panic response to lactate infusion is not confined to panic disorder patients but may relate to baseline anxiety (Cowley *et al.* 1987).

The mechanism producing the panic response to lactate is still not clear despite the extensive research in the area. The influence of carbon dioxide levels, which increase with sodium lactate provoked panic attacks, is one of the proposed mechanisms (Chapter 6) with the possibility that panic disorder patients have a hypersensitivity for inhalation of carbon dioxide. The findings of the Klein group have extended the observations with sodium lactate into the provocation of panic by increased carbon dioxide levels in inhaled air suggesting that an alteration in the physiological setting for overbreathing may be involved in the pathogenesis of panic attacks.

CHOLECYSTOKININ AND PANIC

A promising new approach has been suggested by the findings that a cholecystokinin (CCK) fragment provokes panic in both volunteers, and to a greater extent, in panic disorder patients (Bradwejn *et al.* 1992). This finding suggests the possibility that CCK antagonists might have a role in the treatment of the condition. This work needs to be extended to investigate other related diagnostic groups in order to determine whether this particular reaction and potential therapeutic advance is specific to panic or may affect, as well, those disorders with the closest co-morbid links.

BENZODIAZEPINES AND PANIC

The role of the benzodiazepine receptor in panic disorder has also been extensively investigated using a provocation of panic model (Nutt *et al.* 1990). The interesting finding that benzodiazepine antagonists provoke panic and anxiety, mirrors the finding that treatment of panic disorder patients with benzodiazepines in high doses or with high-potency benzodiazepines is associated with a reduction in panic attacks. From the point of view of treatment, however, the use of high-potency benzodiazepines in the management of panic disorder has problems. Paradoxical aggression and provocation of suicidality reported with benzodiazepines would complicate their use in panic disorder. The development of tolerance, the reactions and rebound anxiety associated with withdrawal are well-known complications of benzodiazepine treatment. Even very slow tapering of doses for withdrawal is not always successful (Fyer *et al.* 1987). Benzodiazepines have a recognized place in short-term use but cannot be regarded as an appropriate choice for the medium or long term.

ANTIDEPRESSANTS, SEROTONIN, AND PANIC DISORDER

The use of antidepressants in the treatment of panic disorder is interesting since conventional doses are often seen to precipitate panic at the start of treatment (Aronson 1987). With low doses however, there are numerous reports of the advantages of antidepressants in panic disorder. In many of the studies that demonstrated efficacy there was, however, a failure to identify or quantify concomitant depression. Since the early reports of the usefulness of imipramine, antidepressants have come to be regarded as the treatment of choice despite the disadvantage of their relatively slow onset of action.

Various antidepressants, both selective or non-selective in their effects on serotonin and noradrenaline receptor systems, have been found to be effective in the treatment of panic disorder. The availability of drugs having selective effects on particular amine systems makes it possible to investigate the possible relative importance of different systems in the disorder.

The consistent reports of the usefulness of clomipramine (Kahn *et al.* 1987; Den Boer and Westenberg 1987; Cassano *et al.* 1988), which has mixed effects but which is a potent serotonin reuptake inhibitor, suggested a possible relationship between serotonin and panic disorder. The reports of the selective efficacy of 5-HT reuptake inhibitors in pure panic without depression compared with other conventional antidepressants, in particular noradrenaline reuptake inhibitors, is interesting in suggesting a selective serotonergic component for pure panic disorder (Den Boer and Westenberg 1988). There is some suggestion of a different pharmacology for the pure panic disorder group compared with those with concomitant depression and this seems to parallel the epidemiological findings that the pure panic group has a different course and morbidity.

Panic disorder patients with concomitant depression appear to have greater morbidity as seen in the social consequences of excess agoraphobia and suicide attempts. Studies in this interesting field will have to take account of these differences and investigate both pure panic disorder and also address the issue of co-morbidity.

REFERENCES

Aronson, T.A. (1987). A naturalistic study of imipramine in panic disorder and agoraphobia. *American Journal of Psychiatry*, **144**, 1014–19.

Bradwejn, J., Koszycki, D., and Shrigui, C. (1991). Enhanced sensitivity to cholecystokinin-tetrapeptide in panic disorder. *Archives of General Psychiatry*, **48**, 603–10.

Cassano, G.B., Petracca, A., and Perugi, G. (1988). Clomipramine for panic disorder I. The first 10 weeks of a long-term comparison with imipramine. *Journal of Affective Disorders*, **14**, 123–27.

Coryell, W., Endicott, J., Andreasen, N.C., Keller, M.B., Clayton, P.J., Hirschfeld,

R.M.A., Scheftner, W.A., and Winokur, G. (1988). Depression and panic attacks: the significance of overlap as reflected in follow-up and family study data. *American Journal of Psychiatry*, **145**, 293–300.

Cowley, D.S., Hyde, T.S., Dager, S.R., and Dunner, D.L. (1987). Lactate infusions: the role of baseline anxiety. *Psychiatry Research*, **21**, 169–79.

Den Boer J.A., Westenberg, H.G.M., Kamerbeek, W.D.J., Verhoeven, W.M.A., and Kahn, R.S. (1987). Effect of serotonin uptake inhibitors in anxiety disorders, a double-blind comparison of clomipramine and fluvoxamine. *International Clinical Psychopharmacology*, **2**, 21–32.

Den Boer, J.A. and Westenberg, H.G. (1988). Effect of a serotonin and noradrenaline uptake inhibitor in panic disorder, a double blind comparative study with fluvoxamine and maprotiline. *International Clinical Psychopharmacology*, **3**, 59–74.

Diagnostic and statistical manual of mental disorders. (1988). American Psychiatric Association, Washington, DC.

Fyer, A.J., Lievowitz, M.R., and Gorman J.M. (1987). Discontinuation of alprazolam treatment in panic patients. *American Journal of Psychiatry*, **144**, 303–8.

Gorman, J.M., Askanazi, J., Liebowitz, M.R., Fyer, A.J., Stein, J., Kinney, J.M., and Klein, D.F. (1984). Response to hyperventilation in a group of patients with panic disorder. *American Journal of Psychiatry*, **141**, 857–61.

Johnson, J., Weissman, M.M., and Klerman, G.L. (1990). Panic disorder, comorbidity, and suicide attempts. *Archives of General Psychiatry*, **47**, 805–8.

Kahn, R.S., Westenberg, H.G.M., Verhoeven, W.M.A., Gispen de Wied, C.C., and Kamerbeek, W.D.J. (1987). Effect of a serotonin precursor and uptake inhibitor in anxiety disorders, a double blind comparison of 5-hydroxytryptophan, clomipramine and placebo. *International Clinical Psychopharmacology*, **2**, 33–45.

Klein, D.F. (1964). Delineation of two drug responsive anxiety syndromes. *Psychopharmacologia*, **5**, 397–408.

Margraf, J., Ehlers, A., and Roth, W.T. (1986). Sodium Lactate and panic attacks: a review and critique. *Psychosomatic Medicine*, **48**, 23–51.

Markowitz, J.S., Weissman, M.M., Ouellette, R., Lish, J.D., and Klerman, G.L. (1989). Quality of life in panic disorder. *Archives of General Psychiatry*, **46**, 984–92.

Nutt, D.J., Glue, P., Lawson, C.W., and Wilson, S. (1990). Flumazenil provocation of panic attacks: evidence for altered benzodiazepine receptor sensitivity in panic disorder. *Archives of General Psychiatry*, **47**, 917–25.

Stein, M.B. and Uhde, T.W. (1988). Panic disorder and major depression. A tale of two syndromes. *Psychiatric Clinics of North America*, **11**, 441–61.

Vollrath, M. and Angst, J. (1989). Outcome of panic and depression in a seven-year follow-up: results of the Zurich study. *Acta Psychiatrica Scandinavica*, **80**, 591–6.

Vollrath, M., Koch, R., and Angst, J. (1990). The Zurich study. IX Panic disorder and sporadic panic: symptoms, diagnosis, prevalence, and overlap with depression. *European Archives of Psychiatry and Neurological Science*, **239**, 221–30.

von Korff, M.R., Eaton, W.W., and Keyl, P.M. (1985). The epidemiology of panic attacks and panic disorder. *American Journal of Epidemiology*, **122**, 970–81.

2

The epidemiology of frequent and less frequent panic attacks

JULES ANGST and WERNER WICKI

INTRODUCTION

The concepts of panic attack and panic disorder are relatively new and still undergoing changes in their definition. Whereas DSM-III and DSM-III-R consider panic disorder as an independent diagnostic entity, it is in ICD-10 subsumed to phobic disorder. In DSM-III-R, several sets of criteria are used for the definition of panic disorder: spontaneity of attacks, frequency of attacks within a certain period of time, the presence of a persistent fear of having another attack. Furthermore, a distinction is made between full panic attacks (4 of 12 or 13 symptoms) and limited symptom attacks (less than 4 symptoms). These criteria were mainly developed by committees of experienced clinical researchers, and only to a limited extent based on empirical data from community studies optimizing the case definition by varying the diagnostic criteria and validating them.

From an epidemiological point of view it is obvious that panic attacks occur frequently in non-clinical subjects of the normal population, and here the distinction between non-cases and cases is not easy to make. There may be a continuum of severity from brief spells of anxiety to severe panic attacks as suggested by Norton et al. (1988).

This chapter tries to contribute to the case definition by presenting data from a relatively small but prospective study from age 20 to 30, carried out in a Swiss cohort of the community. We will describe in a very elementary way the occurrence of panic attacks and their symptoms regardles of the diagnostic threshold. In this way, subjects with only one, or two to three panic attacks over a full year are compared to those with attacks of higher frequency. Comparison is made using traditional validators for diagnosis, for instance, work impairment, treatment rates, family history. Thus, the attempt will be made to vary diagnostic criteria in order to validate them and to contribute to an optimal case definition.

Furthermore some co-morbidity data will be presented which may contribute to the delineation between panic disorder, other anxiety disorders, and depression.

METHODOLOGY

The Zurich study has been described earlier (Angst *et al.* 1984). A cohort of 292 males and 299 females aged 19–20 from the Canton of Zurich in Switzerland was selected, enriched by high scorers on the SCL-90-Hopkins symptom check-list (SCL-90-R, Derogatis 1977). There were four waves of interviews: 1979, 1981, 1986, and 1988. The drop-out rate after the fourth interview wave (10 years after the first interview) was 28 per cent. The data presented are mainly collected during the last interview carried out at age 30 in 1988 in 424 subjects (200 m, 224 f). They are based on all subjects ever interviewed ($N = 591$) taking into account longitudinal data from four interviews from age 20 to 30.

Panic attacks were systematically assessed in a special section of the SPIKE interview at age 28 (1986) and age 30 (1988). The probe question was: 'Did you during the past 12 months suffer from sudden anxiety or panic attacks?' If yes, 'were they totally unexpected or did they occur in certain situations?' In a further step, 25 symptoms (1986) or 16 (1988) of panic attacks were evaluated. In addition, in an open question, further symptoms could be added. The estimated length of attacks to the peak was recorded in minutes in 1988. In addition, frequency and recency of attacks, help-seeking behaviour and social consequences (work or leisure impairment) were assessed. At each interview, the previous history, including age of onset and age of first treatment, was asked about. Also the family history for panic attacks for father, mother, and siblings was noted in 1986. No exclusion criteria were applied.

The diagnosis of panic disorder was made according to DSM-III criteria. In addition under this threshold, a diagnosis of 'sporadic panic' was made which was defined and elaborated on in another paper (Vollrath *et al.* 1990). As DSM-III panic disorder it requires a minimum of 4 of 12 of the symptoms, but only 4 attacks over 12 months are necessary for the case definition. Both groups together, DSM-III panic disorder and sporadic panic, are called 'panic syndromes' or 'panic' in this paper.

A number of other psychiatric diagnoses are based on DSM-III criteria: generalized anxiety disorder, agoraphobia, social phobia, simple phobia, major depressive disorder. Dysthymia is based on DSM-III-R criteria. A further group of syndromes is used for the study of co-morbidity with panic disorder: recurrent brief depression (defined in Angst *et al.* 1990*b*). The criteria for a new diagnostic class of 'recurrent brief anxiety' are

TABLE 2.1. *Diagnostic criteria for recurrent brief anxiety (RBA)*

1. Anxiety, i.e. fear to be alone, fear of misfortune, anxious about the next day.
2. 3 of 4 DSM-III categories of symptoms of GAD.
3. The anxious mood has to be present for 1–13 days with a recurrence of at least once a month in the past year.
4. Subjective work impairment.

TABLE 2.2. *1-Year prevalence rates of panic attacks at age 30*

	males	Weighted rates/100 females	m + f	Sex ratio f : m
Panic attacks	4.8	14.9	10.0	3.1
Spontaneous attacks	1.7	2.3	2.0	1.3
Situational attacks	3.1	12.9	8.1	4.2

listed in Table 2.1. It consists of recurrent brief anxiety states with identical symptoms as generalized anxiety disorder. The syndrome was described in another paper (Angst and Wicki 1992). Some further variables are included in the analyses of co-morbidity: a history of suicide attempts, migraine (Merikangas *et al.* 1990), insomnia (Angst *et al.* 1989), neurasthenia (Angst and Koch 1991). The diagnosis of alcoholism approximates the criteria as given by Guze *et al.* (1986). 'Weight concerns' and 'binge eating' are defined in the paper of Vollrath *et al.* (1992). Sexual dysfunction includes female sexual arousal disorder, male erectile disorder, orgasm disorders, sexual pain disorders. Low sexual desire meets the diagnostic criteria of hypoactive sexual desire disorders of DSM-III-R.

FREQUENCY OF PANIC ATTACKS OVER ONE YEAR AS A DIAGNOSTIC CRITERION

At age 30, 12 of 200 males and 34 of 224 females had suffered from panic attacks over the past 12 months. Twenty per cent of these subjects suffered from spontaneous and 80 per cent from situational attacks (Table 2.2). Weighted back to the normal population, we find a 1-year prevalence rate of panic attacks of 10 per cent (4.8 for males and 14.9 for females). Twenty per cent of them reported spontaneous attacks. Two-point-six per cent suffered from one attack, 2.5 per cent from two to three attacks, and 4.9 per cent from four or more attacks over one year (Table 2.3). In Table

TABLE 2.3. *Panic attacks: unweighted and weighted 1-year rates at age 30*

Number of panic attacks over 1 yr	N cases	Weighted rates/100
1	6	2.6
2–3	15	2.5
4–7	11	2.9
8–11	5	1.4
1–2/month	6	0.3
weekly	4	0.2
All together	47	10.0

TABLE 2.4. *Classification by number of panic attacks (1 year) and its validation*

Panic attacks (1 yr)	1	2–3	4–7	≥ 8
Subjects	6	15	11	15
Criterial symptoms				
DSM-III ($\bar{x}$)	4.0	5.2	5.5	5.9
DSM-III-R ($\bar{x}$)	3.8	5.2	5.5	5.9
Professional treatment (%)				
Panic 1988	17	33	36	27
Panic lifetime	33	53	63	40
Anxiety/Depression lifetime	50	73	73	67
Impairment (%)				
Work	17	47	64	13
Leisure or work	33	80	82	87
Family history (%)				
Panic	17	7	18	13
Anxiety	50	67	45	47
Depression	67	73	73	60
All three	83	87	82	67

2.4 the subjects are classified by the number of panic attacks over one year. The subgroups are then validated by the number of criterial symptoms, treatment rates, impairment rates and family history rates. It is noticeable that the observed number of criterial symptoms listed in the DSM-III or DSM-III-R, do not differ from each other considerably. We prefer the definition of DSM-III, which is stricter. Table 2.4 shows that subjects with only one panic attack differ from those with multiple attacks. It is remarkable that even in subjects with a single panic attack lifetime treatment rates were 33 per cent for panic, and 50 per cent for any anxiety or depressive disorder. Subjects with multiple attacks were treated more frequently (40–63 per cent) and over lifetime over 51 and 70 per cent respectively. Impairment was assessed for the domains of work, personal relationships, and leisure activities. One can recognize that some subjects fell impaired at work, whereas others much more so in other activities. This favours the inclusion of both aspects as criteria for validation. Multiple panickers feel impaired in 80–87 per cent, single attack subjects in only 33 per cent. A positive family history for panic or anxiety among first-degree relatives is not related to the frequency of panic attacks over one year. But the family history for anxiety does distinguish panickers from controls.

Taking all the information of Table 2.4 together, two findings stand out: single attack subjects have fewer symptoms, lower treatment rates, less impairment, but do not differ in a positive family history from the other groups consisting of subjects with multiple attacks. Within the other groups, none of the validators clearly differentiates. (The finding that subjects with weekly attacks give lower family history and lower actual treatment rates is not conclusive in the face of the small number of subjects $\langle N = 4 \rangle$.) On the whole, *subjects with two or more attacks over one year seem to form a rather homogeneous group. From this point of view, a case definition taking into account frequency of panic attacks would require only two attacks over one year as a minimum.*

NUMBER OF SYMPTOMS AS A DIAGNOSTIC CRITERION

DSM-III requires a minimum of 4 of 12 symptoms for the diagnosis of panic disorder. In Table 2.5, the subjects are grouped by the total number of criterial panic symptoms of DSM-III. Nine subjects experienced only 1–3 symptoms and do therefore not meet the threshold for DSM-III panic attack. Twenty-two subjects had 4–6 symptoms and 15 subjects 7–12 symptoms. Subjects with limited symptom attacks (1–3 symptoms) gave a 1-year prevalence rate of 2.8 per cent (males 1.4 per cent, females 4.1 per cent). At least 4 of 12 symptoms were present in 7.1 per cent of the population (m 3.4 per cent, f 10.7 per cent). The symptom threshold chosen by the DSM-III fits the data: subjects with limited attacks defined by the presence of 1–3 symptoms suffer from fewer attacks, are less frequently treated, and considerably less impaired than subjects with DSM-III panic disorder. Again the family history does not differentiate cases from subjects with limited attacks.

Subjects with limited attacks (less than 4 of 12 DSM-III symptoms) accounted for a 1-year prevalence rate of 2.8 per cent, whereas 7.2 per cent for the normal population at age 30 met the symptom criteria.

TABLE 2.5. *Classification by total number of DSM-III panic symptoms and its validation (1988, age 30)*

		Number of DSM-III symptoms			
		0	1–3	4–6	7–12
Subjects	424	371	9	22	15
	N	%	%	%	%
Attacks (1 yr)					
1	6	–	11	14	7
2–3	5	–	33	41	20
4–7	11	–	33	14	33
> 7	15	–	22	31	40
Professional treatment					
Panic 1988	14	0	0	41	33
Panic lifetime	42	5	33	55	53
Social impairment	35	0	22	82	93
Positive family history					
Panic	40	9	11	14	13
Anxiety	117	25	56	50	53

CASE DEFINITION

From the distribution of the previous data it is obvious that the threshold of case definition is arbitrary and that we are dealing with a continuum on both criteria, number of attacks and number of symptoms. The validation of case definition by external criteria (treatment rates, impairment, family history) suggests the following diagnostic criteria for panic disorder:

- minimum number of DSM-III criterial symptoms: 4 of 12 as in DSM-III;

- minimal frequency of panic attacks over 1 year — 2.

This case definition would require even less attacks per year than we suggested in another paper where we used at least four attacks per year for a diagnosis of 'sporadic panic' or infrequent panic (Vollrath *et al.* 1990). In order to remain conservative we shall continue to use the earlier, stricter criterion (four attacks/one year) in this chapter.

LENGTH OF PANIC ATTACKS TO THE PEAK

The length of panic symptoms to the peak of the attacks was assessed at age 30 in 21 subjects. The length reported by the subjects is only a rough

TABLE 2.6. *1-year prevalence rates of diagnoses*

	1986	1988
Panic DSM-III		
males	0.3	1.4
females	0.6	2.1
m + f	0.5	1.7
Sporadic panic		
males	0.2	0.3
females	3.4	3.1
m + f	1.8	1.7
All panic		
males	0.5	1.7
females	4.1	5.2
m + f	2.3	3.5

estimate. Table 2.4 gives the distribution. Twenty-five per cent lasted 1–8 min, another 25 per cent 9–30 min and 50 per cent lasted 1–4 h. The median was 30 min.

ONE-YEAR PREVALENCE RATES OF PANIC DISORDER

DSM-III panic disorder was found in 0.5 per cent at age 28 and in 1.7 per cent at age 30. 'Sporadic panic' (at least 4 panic attacks over 1 year) occured in 1.8 per cent and 1.7 per cent respectively. The female/male ratio is 3:1 (Table 2.6).

ASSOCIATION OF PANIC DISORDERS WITH OTHER PSYCHIATRIC DIAGNOSES OR SYNDROMES

Because no exclusion criteria were applied, we can examine the association of panic with other psychiatric conditions. The association between panic and other psychiatric syndromes was computed in two ways: (1) cross-sectionally over 1 year for the fourth interview carried out at age 30 in 1988, and (2) longitudinally taking into account the diagnoses of two (1986, 1988) or all four interviews (1979, 1981, 1986, 1988). The periods taken into account are indicated in the tables.

Association of panic disorder with other anxiety disorders

Table 2.7 gives the rate of co-occurrence of other diagnoses with panic disorder cross-sectionally at age 30 and longitudinally from age 20 to 30.

TABLE 2.7. *Cross-sectional and longitudinal association of panic with other diagnoses*

	Cross-section			Longitudinal		
	N = 22			N = 96		
	% panic associated with	odds ratio	95% confidence bounds	% panic associated with	odds ratio	95% confidence bounds
General anxiety disorder	4.6	1.6*	0.2–13.7	6.8	1.3*	0.5–3.5
Recurrent brief anxiety	27.3	6.4	2.3–18.1	20.5	3.4	1.8–6.6
Agoraphobia DSM-III	14.3	10.7	3.2–35.5	6.5	5.8	1.7–19.1
Social phobia DSM-III	14.3	5.3	1.3–20.4	5.2	1.6	0.5–5.2
Simple phobia DSM-III	23.8	3.1	1.1–8.5	13.0	1.4	0.6–3.1
Major depression disorder DSM-III	13.6	1.2	0.3–4.5	35.4	1.8	1.1–2.9
Recurrent brief depression	27.3	7.2	2.5–20.2	59.4	5.8	3.6–9.2
Dysthymia DSM-III-R	4.6	2.0	0.2–17.1	13.6	4.4	1.9–10.0
Depression all	10.9	3.6	1.5–8.9	79.2	6.8	4.0–11.5
Suicide attempts	9.1	3.9*	0.8–19.0	24.0	4.2	2.3–7.6
Hypomania	14.3	3.6	0.9–13.7	9.1	1.1*	0.5–2.5
Migraine	40.9	2.3*	0.9–5.4	29.4	2.1	1.2–3.5
Insomnia	63.6	3.7	1.5–9.2	56.8	1.9	1.2–3.0
Neurasthenia	42.9	4.7	1.8–11.7	54.2	3.9	2.5–6.2
Alcoholism	9.5	1.6*	0.5–12.4	14.8	2.5	0.8–7.0
Weight concerns	40.9	1.7*	0.7–4.2	35.4	1.5*	0.9–2.4
Binge eating	22.7	6.6	2.5–17.6	11.5	2.2	1.0–4.6
Sexual dysfunction	19.1	2.5*	0.8–7.8			
Low sexual desire	27.2	2.5*	0.9–6.5			

* p = ns.

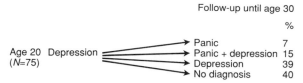

FIG. 2.1. Follow-up of subjects with depression.

Cross-sectionally, simple phobia was found in 23 per cent of panic subjects but longitudinally in only 8 per cent, whereas agoraphobia was present cross-sectionally in 14 per cent and longitudinally in 20 per cent. Social phobia was found infrequently in 14 and 8 per cent respectively. Any phobia was present in 36.4 per cent of panic subjects compared to 11.9 per cent of controls.

The *cross-sectional* association with panic disorder is highest for DSM-III agoraphobia (odds ratio 10.7), followed by recurrent brief anxiety (6.4), and social phobia DSM-III-R (5.3). Simple phobia is significantly associated to a lower extent (odds ratio 3.1). It is interesting that generalized anxiety disorder shows no significant association with panic disorder, whereas the recurrent brief subtype of anxiety is strongly associated. From a clinical point of view this association makes sense.

Longitudinally neither generalized anxiety disorders nor social phobia are associated significantly with panic disorder. Again agoraphobia shows the highest odds ratio (5.8) followed by recurrent brief anxiety (3.4).

Association with depression

Table 2.7 shows that cross-sectionally 41 per cent of panic subjects suffered from depression in the same year and that the rate increased longitudinally to 79 per cent. Most frequently present was recurrent brief depression with a presence of 27 per cent cross-sectionally and 59 per cent longitudinally, followed by major depression with a rate of 14 per cent cross-sectionally and 35 per cent longitudinally (Fig. 2.1). It is surprising that DSM-III major depressive disorder is neither cross-sectionally nor longitudinally strongly associated with panic disorder, whereas dysthymia and recurrent brief depression are. The association of dysthymia increases from the cross-sectional (2.0) to the longitudinal approach (4.4). But recurrent brief depression is more strongly associated with panic disorder cross-sectionally (7.2) and longitudinally (5.8).

The considerable association of panic disorder with dysthymia and recurrent brief depression deserves further longitudinal analysis, taking into account age of onset of panic and depression (see Chapter 10).

Association of panic disorder with other diagnoses

The association of panic disorder with depression on one hand and the association of depression with suicide attempts, neurasthenia, and insomnia on the other (Merikangas *et al.*, in press) suggests that some of these syndromes should also be associated with panic disorder. This is confirmed by the data in Table 2.7. The highest association with panic disorder is found for neurasthenia, followed by insomnia and suicide attempts. Hypomania is only associated cross-sectionally to a significant degree (odds ratio 3.6), whereas the longitudinal association is non-significant. This result may be explained by the relatively late diagnosis of hypomania made in this study on the occasion of the last two interviews at age 28 and 30. Migraine is inconsistently associated whereas alcoholism is not associated to a significant extent with panic disorder in this young cohort. This does not exclude a future association after a longer lasting course of panic disorder. It is interesting that binge eating as another highly recurrent syndrome is associated with panic disorder, especially cross-sectionally with an odds ratio of 6.6.

Association of panic disorder with agoraphobia and suicide attempts controlling for depression

Thompson *et al.* (1989) described the lack of association between panic disorder and agoraphobia in a community study where panic patients did not suffer from depression.

A more detailed analysis of panic subjects with and without major depressive disorder compared to subjects with major depression without panic, and controls is given in Table 2.8. It gives the frequency of agoraphobia and suicide attempts in all four groups. In controls and pure major depressives we found only 2.6 and 2.8 per cent agoraphobics. In subjects with pure panic the figure was 7.4 per cent and in subjects with panic and major depressive disorder it was 28.6 per cent. The only group which has a tenfold higher association with agoraphobia is the group of panic subjects suffering from major depression too. In the lower part of Table 2.8 a similar analysis is carried out for panic subjects with and without any diagnosis of depression (major depressive disorder, recurrent brief depression, dysthymia). Again the association between panic and agoraphobia is mainly present in subjects with both panic and any diagnosis of depression. Unfortunately, the numbers are too small for statistical comparisons.

The breakdown of panic subjects with and without depression is more interesting in regard of the presence of suicide attempts. Suicide attempts are threefold more frequent in pure panic subjects and even eightfold more frequent in subjects with both panic and depression, than in controls. If we

TABLE 2.8. *Association of panic with agoraphobia and suicide attempts by presence or absence of major depression (MDD) or any diagnosis (Dx) of depression (RBD, MDD, Dysthymia)*

	Controls	Panic without MDD	Panic with MDD	MDD without panic	p
Subjects (8688)[1]	351	27	14	72	
Agoraphobia (%)	2.6	7.4	28.6	2.8	–
Subjects[2]	382	62	34	113	
Suicide attempters (%)	4.5	16.1	38.2	15.0	0.001

	Controls	Panic without depression Dx	Panic with depression Dx	Depression without panic	p
Subjects (8688)	301	14	27	122	
Agoraphobia (%)	3.0	7.1	18.5	1.6	–
Subjects	318	20	76	177	
Suicide attempters (%)	3.5	5.0	28.9	13.0	0.001

[1] 8688 = sample 1986 and 1988 (N = 462).
[2] Total sample 1979 (N = 591).

TABLE 2.9. *Primary and secondary panic in cases of co-morbidity (N = 76)* *(Defined by age of onset of symptoms)*

| | 10-year rates/100 | |
	Unweighted	Weighted
Primary panic (PAN → DEP)	2.0	1.06
Secondary panic (DEP → PAN)	6.9	5.0
Simultaneous onset	0.3	0.06

define again depression by the presence of MDD, RBD, or dysthymia, then panic subjects without any diagnosis of depression do not differ clearly in the rate of suicide attempters (5 per cent) from controls (3.5 per cent). Among depressives without panic we find a suicide attempt rate of 13 per cent, the co-morbid group (panic with depression) has a rate of 28.9 per cent. It is known that subjects with RBD have a relatively pronounced suicide attempt rate. Furthermore, RBD is highly associated with panic disorder and seems to explain a large number of suicide attempts among panic subjects.

Table 2.8 shows how important it is to distinguish between panic alone and panic with depression, the latter not only defined as major depression but also as recurrent brief depression.

PRIMARY AND SECONDARY PANIC

The question, 'What is first, panic or depression?' is difficult to analyse. The easiest approach seems to be based on age of onset. But data on age of onset are retrospective and therefore not very reliable. For a diagnosis it is even more difficult to collect reliable data required in retrospect. Furthermore subjects who may meet, at a certain age, criteria for a diagnosis, may show a much earlier onset of symptoms. The best answer would be given by data collected prospectively. This is almost unfeasable in a cohort of the normal population. The authors will now present their results based on age of onset of symptoms and based on prospectively collected interview diagnoses.

In Table 2.9 76 probands with both the diagnoses, panic disorder and major depression, or recurrent brief depression, are subclassified by *age of onset of symptoms* into primary and secondary panic. Nine-point-two per cent of the subjects met diagnostic criteria for both the diagnoses, panic and depression over 10 years. The unweighted rate of subjects with primary panic was 2.0 per cent, whereas the remaining 6.9 per cent devel-

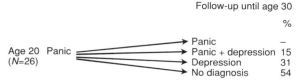

FIG. 2.2. Follow-up of subjects with panic.

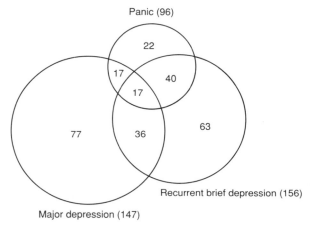

FIG. 2.3. Overlap of panic with major depression and recurrent brief depression.

oped panic secondary to depression; very few had a simultaneous onset. Weighted back to the normal population we find a *10-year prevalence rate of only 1 per cent for primary panic and 5 per cent for secondary panic.* These figures refer to cases with co-morbidity with depression.

This finding is astonishing: the usual data in the literature, and our own earlier data based on diagnoses, suggest that panic is not stable but develops frequently into depression (Angst *et al*. 1990*a*). This is now again confirmed by our follow-up until age 30 of subjects first diagnosed with depression (*N* = 75) or panic (*N* = 26) at age 20. Very few depressives only developed panic later (7 per cent), a minority both panic and depression (15 per cent), whereas the majority suffered from depression again (39 per cent) or recovered (40 per cent) (Fig. 2.2). On the other hand none of the 26 panic subjects remained a pure panic disorder. Fifteen per cent suffered later simultaneously or subsequently from both depression and panic, 31 per cent from depression, and only 23 per cent recovered during the follow-up period until age 30 (Fig. 2.3).

This data suggests very strongly that longitudinally on a diagnostic level, a majority of subjects with panic develop depression, while a minority recovers to a certain extent.

DISCUSSION

The sample used in this study is enriched by risk cases for psychiatric syndromes due to the over-representation of high scorers on the SCL-90-R (Angst *et al.* 1984). However, by weighting back to the normal population true prevalence rates can be computed.

At age 30, panic attacks were found in 10 per cent of the normal population with a sex ratio of 3:1 in favour of females. This rate is more or less identical with the one from the Munich study published by Wittchen (1986) who found a prevalence rate of 9.3 per cent (males 7.1 per cent, females 11.1 per cent), and also similar to the prevalence of a history of panic attacks of 10 per cent described by von Korff *et al.* (1985) for the ECA study. Salge *et al.* (1988) found in another community study a prevalence rate of panic attacks of 14.1 per cent (11 per cent males, 15.8 per cent females). Joyce *et al.* (1989) report a lifetime prevalence rate of 7.8 per cent (2.2 per cent males, 11.3 per cent females). Based on the community studies, we can assume a one-year prevalence rate for panic attacks of about 10 per cent in the community. (In contrast to these figures, which are based on interviews, questionnaire studies of non-representative student samples give much higher rates varying from 34 per cent (Norton *et al.* 1988) to 35.9 per cent (Norton *et al.* 1986). Also Margraf and Ehlers (1988) found in two other studies of students at least equally high rates.) Every fifth panic subject experienced spontaneous attacks, a figure which is comparable to the 16.4 per cent reported by Salge *et al.* (1988). But the distinction between spontaneous and situational panic attacks is difficult to make and according to Gelder (1988) unlikely to be valid.

There is not much data from community studies on subthreshold panic syndromes.

The authors' attempt to validate several diagnostic thresholds by subdividing panic subjects by number of attacks over one year and number of symptoms experienced, suggests the exclusion of subjects with one attack only, but the inclusion of all subjects with more than one attack. Persons with few or multiple attacks do not differ in frequency of symptoms, impairment, treatment rates, or family history. The threshold of 4 of 12 symptoms required for a diagnosis of panic disorder (DSM-III) is clearly supported by our data. The adding of a thirteenth symptom by DSM-III-R seems to be unnecessary and redundant.

Subjects with limited panic attacks (suffering from less than 4 of 12

DSM-III criterial symptoms for panic disorder) form a milder affected group which does require further research, especially follow-up studies. These subjects may be at risk for developing later panic disorder. The authors found a 1-year prevalence rate of limited panic attacks of 2.8 per cent (males 1.4 per cent, females 4.1 per cent). This figure would be comparable to a frequency published by Korff *et al.* (1985) of the ECA study given for 6 months and mentioning a prevalence for DSM-III panic disorder between 0.6 and 1.0 per cent, for recurrent and severe attacks between 0.8 and 1.0 per cent, and for single panic attacks between 1 and 1.4 per cent. All figures add up to about 3 per cent over 6 months. In the study of Norton *et al.* (1988) of college students, there was a relatively high frequency of subjects with limited panic symptoms. They comprised about one-fifth of the panickers.

On a diagnostic level the authors did not apply any exclusion criteria in order to be able to examine the association between panic and other psychiatric syndromes. DSM-III panic disorder showed a 1-year prevalence rate of 0.5 per cent at age 28 and 1.7 per cent at age 30. These figures are comparable with those of the literature. Weissman *et al.* (1988) report a point prevalence of 0.4 per cent in the New Haven study and a 6-month prevalence rate of 0.6–1.0 per cent for the ECA study. Uhlenhuth *et al.* (1983) found a 1-year prevalence rate of 1.2 per cent. The lifetime prevalence rates vary between 1.2 per cent (Bland *et al.* 1988) and 2–3 per cent (Lehtinen 1989) to 2–4 per cent (Wittchen 1986). The female/male ratio in this study is about 2 : 1.

In addition the authors diagnosed, as described in an earlier paper (Vollrath *et al.* 1990), a group of subjects with 'sporadic panic' defined by the presence of at least four typical panic attacks over one year. The 1-year prevalence rate is about the same as for panic disorder. In the following, the authors have unified DSM-III panic disorder and sporadic panic disorder as 'panic syndromes' or 'panic'.

The authors' analysis of the association between panic syndromes and other psychiatric syndromes is intended to contribute to the question of the independent existence of panic. The conclusions are based on cross-sectional associations over 1 year at age 30 and longitudinal associations over 10 years (from age 20 to 30).

The majority of panic subjects did not receive another diagnosis of anxiety disorder. Thirty-six per cent of panic subjects suffered from some kind of phobic disorder compared to 12 per cent among the controls. The association with panic was highest for agoraphobia (odds ratio 10.7), but one has to be aware that only six of 41 (15 per cent) panic subjects suffered from agoraphobia. Thompson *et al.* (1989) found co-morbidity of agoraphobia with panic disorder only in the presence of depression. In our data there is a trend to this direction: 7.4 per cent of panic subjects without major depressive disorders had agoraphobia, but in subjects with both panic and major depression 28.6 per cent suffered from agoraphobia. Compared to controls (2.6 per cent) agoraphobia is not over-represented in major depressive disorder (2.8 per cent). Unfortunately, our group of agoraphobics is too small for statistical computations. Therefore, our data can only suggest further investigations.

It is important to notice that there is no significant association between panic and generalized anxiety disorder. Family studies of panic disorder patients do not show an increased rate of GAD (Crowe *et al.* 1983). This finding does not support the hypothesis of a continuum between the two groups.

An outstanding finding is the association of panic with a recurrent brief syndrome of anxiety (recurrent brief anxiety) and with recurrent brief depression and with dysthymia, whereas the overlap with major depressive disorder was considerably lower and cross-sectionally not even significant. A major proportion of dysthymics are recurrent brief depressives and therefore their association is mainly explained by recurrent brief psychiatric syndromes, which have an unpredictable attack-like course pattern as panic has. The finding shows that restricting diagnosis to a minimal length and not considering periodicity is questionable. The link between panic disorder, generalized anxiety disorder and major depressive disorder is negligible compared to the link with recurrent brief anxiety and recurrent brief depression. It is also remarkable that the association of panic with lifetime suicide attempt is mainly given in the presence of depression. Of panic subjects, 23 out of 96 had made a suicide attempt, 22 of the 23 had a diagnosis of depression. Therefore, co-morbidity with depression is extremely important for the analysis of association with other syndromes like agoraphobia or suicide attempts. The findings of Thompson *et al.* (1989) are partially confirmed by the authors'. The link between panic disorder and binge-eating deserves further research and needs replication by other studies. The association of panic with alcoholism is relatively low, but significant (odds ratio 2.5). The study of George *et al.* (1989) would suggest an increasing association with longer follow-up. The close association of panic with neurasthenia is not surprising in the face of the overlap between neurasthenia and depression.

The authors' longitudinal analysis based on age of onset of symptoms or of diagnosis, gives controversial results. Depressive symptoms usually precede panic disorder. But on a diagnostic level, depression only rarely develops into panic (7 per cent). Depression is rather frequently complicated by secondary panic attacks (15 per cent). Depression remains more frequently stable than panic, or takes a favourable course and does not reoccur anymo . Surprisingly, the panic diagnosis did not remain stable at all over 10 years. Panic attacks either disappeared or developed into depression (1/3), or became complicated by depression (15 per cent). The longitudinal analysis is not conclusive, because the data based on age of onset of symptoms are not collected prospectively, and even the prospectively made diagnosis cannot exclude other diagnoses in retrospect. The only conclusion, which can be drawn, is that there is a close link between depression and panic as suggested by Thompson *et al.* (1989). The occurrence of isolated panic is certainly rare. The authors' 10-year prevalence rate is 1 per cent, compared to 5 per cent for secondary panic. More studies are needed on this majority of cases.

ACKNOWLEDGEMENTS

Project supported by grant 3.873.0.88 from the Swiss National Science Foundation.

REFERENCES

Angst, J. and Koch, R. (1991). Neurasthenia in young adults. In *Problems of psychiatry in general practice* (eds M. Gastpar and P. Kielholz), pp. 37–48. Hogrefe & Huber, Lewiston.

Angst, J. and Wicki, W. (1992). The Zurich study. XIII. Recurrent brief anxiety. *European Archives of Psychiatry and Clinical Neuroscience*, **241**, 296–300.

Angst, J., Dobler-Mikola, A., and Binder, J. (1984). The Zurich Study. A prospective epidemiological study of depressive, neurotic and psychosomatic syndromes. I. Problem, methodology. *European Archives of Psychiatry and Neurological Science*, **234**, 13–20.

Angst, J., Vollrath, M., Koch, R., and Dobler-Mikola, A. (1989). The Zurich Study. VII. Insomnia: symptoms, classification and prevalence. *European Archives of Psychiatry and Neurological Science*, **238**, 285–93.

Angst, J., Merkiangas, K., Scheidegger, P., and Wicki, W. (1990*a*). Recurrent brief depression: a new subtype of affective disorder. *Journal of Affective Disorders*, **19**, 87–98.

Angst, J., Vollrath, M., Merikangas, K., and Ernst, C. (1990*b*). Comorbidity of anxiety and depression in the Zurich cohort study of young adults. In *Comorbidity of mood and anxiety disorders*, (eds J.D. Maser and C.R. Cloninger), pp. 123–37. American Psychiatric Press, Washington, DC.

Bland, R.C., Orn, H., and Newman, S.C. (1988). Lifetime prevalence of psychiatric disorders in Edmonton. *Acta Psychiatrica Scandinavica*, **77** (Suppl. 338) 24–32.

Crowe, R.R., Noyes, R., Pauls, D.L., and Slymen, D. (1983). A family study of panic disorder. *Archives of General Psychiatry*, **40**, 1065–9

Derogatis, L.R. (1977). SCL-90. Administration, scoring and procedures. Manual for the R (revised) version and other instruments of the Psychopathology Rating Scale Series. Johns Hopkins University School of Medicine, Baltimore.

Gelder, M.G. (1989). Panic disorder: fact or fiction? *Psychological Medicine*, **19**, 277–83.

George, D.T., Nutt, D.J., Dwyer, B.A., and Linnoila, M. (1990). Alcoholism and panic disorder: is the comorbidity more than coincidence? *Acta Psychiatrica Scandinavica*, **81**, 97–107.

Guze, S.B., Cloninger, C.R., Martin, R., and Clayton, P.J. (1986). Alcoholism as a medical disorder. *Comprehensive Psychiatry*, **27**, 501–10.

Joyce, P.R., Bushnell, J.A., Oakley-Browne, M.A., Wells, J.E., and Hornblow, A.R. (1989). The epidemiology of panic symptomatology and agoraphobic avoidance. *Comprehensive Psychiatry*, **30**, 303–12.

Korff, M.R. von, Eaton, W.W., and Keyl, P.M. (1985). The epidemiology of panic attacks and panic disorder. Results of three community surveys. *American Journal of Epidemiology*, **122**, 970–81.

Lehtinen, V. (1989). Epidemiology of panic disorder. In *Many faces of panic disorder* (eds K. Achte, T. Tamminen and R. Laaksonen), pp. 11–17. *Psychiatria Fennica (Suppl.)*.

Margraf, J. and Ehlers, A. (1988). Panic attacks in nonclinical subjects. In *Panic and phobias II*. (eds I. Hand and H.U. Wittchen), pp. 103–16. Springer, Berlin.

Merikangas, K., Angst, J., and Isler, H. (1990). Migraine and psychopathology. Results of the Zurich cohort study of young adults. *Archives of General Psychiatry*, **47**, 849–53.

Merikangas, K., Wicki, W., and Angst, J. (1992). Heterogeneity of depression: classification of depressive subtypes by longitudinal course. *British Journal of Psychiatry*. (In press.)

Norton, G.R., Cairns, S.L., Wozney, K.A., and Malan, J. (1988). Panic attacks and psychopathology in nonclinical panickers. *Journal of Anxiety Disorders*, **2**, 319–31.

Norton, G.R., Dorward, J., and Cox, B.J. (1986). Factors associated with panic attacks in nonclinical subjects. *Behavior Therapy*, **17**, 239–52.

Salge, R.A., Beck, J.G., and Logan, A.G. (1988). A community survey of panic. *Journal of Anxiety Disorders*, **2**, 157–67.

Thompson, A.H., Bland, R.C., and Orn, H.T. (1989). Relationship and chronology of depression, agoraphobia, and panic disorder in the general population. *Journal of Nervous and Mental Disease*, **177**, 456–63.

Uhlenhuth, E.H., Balter, M.B., Mellinger, G.D., Cisin, I.H., Clinthorne, J. (1983). Symptom checklist syndromes in the general population. Correlations with psychotherapeutic drug use. *Archives of General Psychiatry*, **40**, 1167–73.

Vollrath, M., Koch, R., and Angst, J. (1990). The Zurich Study. IX. Panic disorder and sporadic panic: symptoms, diagnosis, prevalence, and overlap with depression. *European Archives of Psychiatry and Neurological Science*, **239**, 221–30.

Vollrath, M., Koch, R., and Angst, J. (1992). Binge eating and weight concerns among young adults. *British Journal of Psychiatry*, **160**, 498–503.

Weissman, M.M., Leaf, P.J., Tischler, G.L., Blazer, D.G., Karno, M., Livingston Bruce, M., and Florio, L. (1988). Affective disorders in five United States communities. *Psychological Medicine*, **18**, 141–53.

Wittchen, H.U. (1986). Epidemiology of panic attacks and panic disorders. In *Panic and phobias. Empirical evidence of theoretical models and longterm effects of behavioral treatments* (eds I. Hand and H.U. Wittchen), pp. 18–28.

3

Epidemiology of panic

ANDREW C. BRIGGS and R. FIONA STIRTON

INTRODUCTION

Narrowly defined, epidemiology is the study of the distribution of diseases and disorders in a population. It not only involves such indices as incidence and prevalence but also concerns the description of the characteristics of those individuals with a disorder, the identification of risk factors, prevention and even treatment approaches (e.g. the consideration of the characteristics of those who do or do not respond to particular treatments).

The incidence rate measures the number of new cases of a disorder occurring in a given time period. The prevalence rate measures the number of individuals with the disorder within a particular time period, including ongoing and new cases. Prevalence is therefore a function of the incidence and the duration of the disorder.

In the study of psychiatric epidemiology it is necessary to work at symptom or syndromal level. Epidemiology, taxonomy, and classification have mutually supportive roles to play. Classification is dependent on epidemiological data and epidemiologists require adequate classifications at syndromal level to select populations for study.

Within the broad rubric of epidemiology come naturalistic studies, follow-up studies, and pharmacological studies (these can assist in both classification and in generating ideas for further epidemiological studies). Some of these types of studies will be discussed in more detail below.

Panic is a common symptom, occurring on its own or in combination with other symptoms in other disorders. Panic attacks affect some 10 per cent of the population, are troublesome in about 5 per cent and reach the criteria for panic disorder in 2 per cent (Brandon 1989).

EPIDEMIOLOGICAL STUDIES

Panic disorder was not officially recognized as a separate diagnostic entity until 1980 when it was first included in the third edition of the *Diagnostic* and Statistical Manual of Mental Disorders (DSM-III, APA 1980). Therefore, studies of the prevalence of anxiety disorders conducted before this date are likely to have included some panic disorder sufferers within other anxiety disorder groups. Studies conducted since 1980 also use slightly different diagnostic criteria, different types of study populations and varying time scales. This makes direct comparisons between studies difficult.

Agras and colleagues (1969) interviewed 325 people in the United States, including some children, randomly selected from households in the Greater Burlington area. The interview was based on fear questionnaires and looked at 40 commonly feared situations. The 1-year prevalence rates were 7.47 per cent for mildly disabling phobias and 0.22 per cent for severely disabling phobias. Study psychiatrists considered 0.6 per cent to be agoraphobic.

Marks and Lader (1973) reviewed a number of population studies carried out in the United States, Britain, and Sweden. The prevalence of anxiety states ranged from 2 to 5 per cent of the populations studied and were especially common in women aged 16–40.

In the New Haven study (Weissman et al. 1978) 511 people were randomly selected from the general population and interviewed using SADS-L, which generated Research Diagnostic Criteria. They found 1-month prevalence rates of 2.5 per cent for generalized anxiety, 0.4 per cent for panic disorder, and 1.4 per cent for phobic disorder. All the disorders were more common in women than men. Interestingly, they also noted that only 25 per cent of people with anxiety disorders had received any psychiatric help in the last year.

In the National Drug study (Uhlenhuth et al. 1983) a symptom check-list was administered to over 3000 subjects. This study produced DSM-III diagnostic counterparts, although the diagnoses were less reliable because they were raised from symptom check-lists. They found a 1-year prevalence of generalized anxiety of 6.4 per cent. Agoraphobia with panic attacks was reported by 1.2 per cent of the population, and the prevalence of all other phobias was 2.3 per cent. The male to female ratio for agoraphobia with panic attacks was approximately 1 : 3.5.

In the Zurich Study, Angst and Dobler-Mikola (1985) screened more than 6000 young adults using a self rated check-list. A sample of 591 was studied prospectively by means of self rating scales and a structured interview, generating approximated DSM-III diagnoses. Considering here only those people whose symptoms resulted in social impairment or avoidance behaviour, the study found 1-year prevalence rates for generalized anxiety of 5.2 per cent, for panic attacks of 3.1 per cent and for agoraphobia of 2.5 per cent. Panic attacks were 6 times more prevalent in women than men. In the follow-up study of these subjects, 1-year prevalence rates for DSM-III panic disorder are reported of between 0.5 per cent and 0.9 per cent (Vollrath and Angst 1989).

The Epidemiologic Catchment Area survey (ECA, Regier *et al.* 1984) looked at more than 15 000 subjects from the general populations of five American towns. DSM-III diagnoses were again used in this study. This study found 6-month prevalence rates of panic disorder of 0.6–1 per cent and of agoraphobia of 2.7–5.8 per cent. Again, the rates of panic disorder and agoraphobia were higher in women (Weissman 1990).

Surtees and Sashidharan (1986) conducted a community study of women in Edinburgh using a semi-structured interview (Psychiatric Assessment Schedule) and then applied Research Diagnostic Criteria over a limited range of disorders. They found a 1-month prevalence of panic disorder of 0.3 per cent and of generalized anxiety disorder of 4.2 per cent in their sample.

In Florence psychiatrically trained general practitioners administered a structured interview which generated DSM-III/DSM-III-R (APA 1987) diagnoses to 1110 people registered with 6 GPs (Faravelli *et al.* 1989). They found current prevalence rates of 0.27 per cent for agoraphobia, 0.72 per cent for agoraphobia with panic attacks, 2.79 per cent for generalized anxiety disorder, and 0.27 per cent for panic disorder. The female to male ratios were 3:1 for agoraphobia, 7:3 for agoraphobia with panic attacks and 14:1 for panic disorder. Of those subjects who had received a diagnosis of an anxiety disorder 62 per cent had consulted their GP and 50 per cent had consulted a psychiatrist.

Taking into account the different methods used, the presence or absence of diagnostic hierarchies, varying diagnostic criteria, and the different time scales that were used, the results of these studies are reasonably consistent. The prevalence figures for generalized anxiety range from 2 per cent to 6 per cent. For panic disorder the prevalence is between 0.3 per cent and 3 per cent and for agoraphobia it is between 0.3 per cent and 6 per cent. All the studies agree that women suffer from anxiety disorders more frequently than men.

CRITERIA

The studies undertaken in Leicester, and described below, used modified DSM-III/DSM-III-R criteria for diagnosis of panic disorder. Trained interviewers, who were experienced psychiatrists, used the SCID-UP (Structured Clinical Interview for DSM-III — Upjohn Version, Spitzer and Williams 1983) to obtain information on the course of the disorder, and to place subjects into diagnostic categories.

Panic disorder was diagnosed on the presence of discrete episodes or attacks where the subject felt suddenly frightened or experienced extreme discomfort in situations in which most people would not. Some of these episodes had to occur unexpectedly in situations that the subject did not expect to make him or her anxious. During the attacks, the subject must have experienced at least 4 symptoms from a list of 14. These symptoms were: shortness of breath; choking or smothering sensations; palpitations or accelerated heart rate; chest pain or discomfort; sweating; faintness; dizziness, light-headedness or unsteady feelings; nausea or abdominal distress; depersonalization or derealization; numbness or tingling sensations; flushes or chills; trembling or shaking; fear of dying; fear of going crazy or doing something uncontrolled. Most of the symptoms had to be experienced within 10 mins of the onset of the attack. Attacks had to occur at the frequency of at least 1 attack per week for 3 consecutive weeks. Organic causes were excluded.

A positive diagnosis of panic disorder was then subtyped according to the presence or absence of agoraphobic avoidance behaviour, and its severity. Uncomplicated panic disorder was diagnosed where there was no significant avoidance behaviour or fear of situations. Panic disorder with limited phobic avoidance was diagnosed where subjects did not avoid situations but endured them with dread, or where avoidance behaviour was less than that categorized as panic disorder with extensive phobic avoidance, where the subject experienced generalized travel restrictions, a markedly altered life-style, or often needed a companion to assist him or her with going out.

Diagnostic hierarchies were not used, allowing overlapping diagnoses to be made. Other diagnoses which could be made using the SCID-UP were: simple phobia; social phobia; obsessive compulsive disorder; current and past major depressive disorder, with and without melancholia; mania; dysthymia; cyclothymia; psychotic symptoms. Details of the course of the disorder were obtained, and ages of onset and duration for all the main diagnostic categories.

The minimum data collected on any individual was the SCID-UP. However, further data was obtained according to whether the subject was part of the Community Survey, the follow-up study, or entered into Phase II of the Cross-National Collaborative Panic Study comparing the short-term efficacy of imipramine, alprazolam, or placebo in the treatment of panic disorder. The additional measures and instruments will be mentioned later as appropriate.

THE LEICESTER COMMUNITY SURVEY OF PANIC ATTACKS AND PANIC DISORDER

The aims of this study were to establish whether panic disorder could be identified in a British population using the American criteria; to calculate the prevalence of panic attacks and panic disorder in this population; to examine the demographic characteristics of people with these problems; and to identify possible unmet need for treatment. The method used is described in more detail elsewhere (Stirton and Brandon 1988).

An age–sex stratified sample was randomly selected from the age–sex register of a Leicester group general practice. Altogether, 3000 subjects aged between 18 and 65 were sent an explanatory letter and a questionnaire. Up to two reminders were sent to those who did not reply. From the questionnaires returned those people with possible panic attacks were identified by looking at the responses to panic screening questions (derived from the SCID-UP). Potential panickers were then given a short, semi-structured interview over the telephone or during a visit to their home to determine whether they were experiencing panic attacks. If panic attacks were diagnosed, the SCID-UP interview was then administered in order to establish a clear diagnosis of panic disorder. At this stage the subjects were offered treatment if considered appropriate. A sample of the non-responders was interviewed to check whether they differed from the responders in any way. In fact, the non-responders were essentially the same as the responders with regard to all the demographic variables considered and with regard to the prevalence of panic attacks.

Almost a half (48.9 per cent) of the total sample of 3000 replied to the questionnaire. By interviewing those people whose questionnaire response suggested they may be experiencing panic attacks, 24 (3.7 per cent) of the men and 84 (10.3 per cent) of the women were found to have had at least one panic attack in the month before the interview, giving a combined figure of 7.4 per cent of the responders having experienced a panic attack within the last month.

When given the longer SCID-UP interview, 9 (1.4 per cent) of the men and 39 (4.8 per cent) of the women were diagnosed as having panic disorder reaching the modified DSM-III/DSM-III-R criteria. This produces a combined figure of 3.3 per cent for the 1-month prevalence of panic disorder in this particular practice. The study therefore demonstrated that it was possible to identify a group of people suffering from panic disorder, as defined in DSM-III-R (pink draft), in this British population. It also confirms that panic attacks and panic disorder are about 3 times more common in women than men. These figures are in reasonable agreement with the studies discussed above, given the slightly different criteria and groupings (as diagnostic hierarchies were not employed in this study agoraphobic subjects were included in the panic disorder group if they reached the panic disorder criteria).

The results were analysed (using χ^2 and residual analysis) for differences in the distribution of age-groups, marital status, social class and economic position between three groups; (1) those with panic disorder, (2) those with panic attacks but not panic disorder and (3) those with neither panic

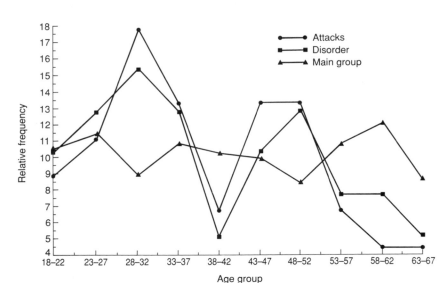

FIG. 3.1. Age group by diagnosis (females).

attacks nor disorder. Unfortunately, racial origin was not included in the study although it is known that this population is predominantly white.

Figure 3.1 shows the relative frequency of women in each age group for the three subpopulations. There is a bimodal age distribution in both of the panic groups which is not merely a reflection of the age distribution of the underlying population. Although not reaching a level of statistical significance this interesting finding warrants further investigation and may reflect periods in life when changes in supportive relationships are especially likely to occur. In men any pattern in age distribution is not obvious but the numbers in the two panic groups are small.

There was a significant difference ($p < 0.001$) in the marital status of the three groups. Both men and women who were divorced or separated were over-represented in the panic attack group. This is similar to the findings of the ECA study (von Korff *et al.* 1985). The economic position of the three groups was considered, that is whether they were working, unemployed, off sick, housewives, retired and so on. For women, there was a significant difference between the three groups, with unemployed women and housewives over represented in the panic disorder group ($p < 0.001$). Although there was a trend for a higher proportion of men with panic attacks or disorder to be unemployed, this did not reach a level of significance.

There was no significant difference in the distribution of social class in men or women, although there does appear to be a trend for lower social classes to be over represented in the panic groups.

When comparing the frequency distributions of the demographic variables it emerged that the group with panic attacks was more similar to the panic disorder group than the no panic group. This is also in keeping with recent research findings (von Korff *et al.* 1985).

It has often been stated that panic disorder sufferers are a serious drain on resources, presenting to many other specialties and incurring expensive investigations before reaching more appropriate treatment agencies. Psychiatric or psychological treatment can be time consuming and there-fore relatively expensive but is often effective for this group of patients. All of these factors must be weighed against the costs of time lost from work and the emotional costs to the sufferers and their families.

Of the panic disorder group, 10 were already receiving treatment when interviewed. Five more accepted treatment as a result of the study contact, but 33 did not want treatment or it was not felt to be necessary. However, it was noted that some of those who declined treatment had seriously limited life-styles because of their symptoms (i.e. were house-bound or unable to work). Usually people in this group stated that they had made satisfactory arrangements with friends or relatives which allowed them to cope with their symptoms. However, they were grateful to have knowledge of the treatments available in case their circumstances changed.

PANIC DISORDER CLINIC

In addition to the Community Survey, a Panic Disorder Clinic was set up, accepting patients referred from general practitioners, psychiatrists, and psychologists, for assessment and advice on treatment. In total, 190 patients with panic disorder have been documented, and a further 18 suffer panic attacks but do not fulfill all the criteria for the disorder. The most common reason for subjects with panic attacks failing to reach disorder criteria is that the attacks are infrequent ($N = 15$). A number of these suffer from agoraphobia and would, therefore, now fulfill the current DSM-III-R criteria ($N = 8$).

Three different aspects of the results from this sample will be described here. These are, firstly, the sex differences between subtypes; secondly, the ages of onset of panic attacks, panic disorder and agoraphobic avoid-ance across subtypes; and, thirdly, the diagnoses which overlap with panic disorder in this sample.

Sex differences

Overall, the male/female ratio in the sample was 0.4. The ratios for the three subtypes of panic disorder — uncomplicated, with limited phobic avoidance, and with extensive phobic disorder — were, respectively, 0.8, 0.4, and 0.04. Indeed, only two men were placed in the category of panic disorder with extensive phobic avoidance. There is a clear sex difference, with women displaying more agoraphobic avoidance than men. However, there is very little sex difference for uncomplicated panic disorder.

Ages of onset

Most patients were able to date the onset of various problems to within a few months, and they quite clearly distinguished between onset of simple and social phobias, panic attacks, frequent and troublesome panic attacks (panic disorder), agoraphobia, and depression. The ages of onset of panic attacks, panic disorder, and agoraphobia for the three subtypes are shown in Table 3.1.

An overwhelming majority (95 per cent) of patients with agoraphobia gave a good description of panic attacks occurring before any avoidance behaviour, and many thought that the panics had led to agoraphobia. This confirms the American viewpoint proposed by Klein (1981) and embodied in DSM-III-R, that agoraphobia is a complication of a primary panic disorder. Of interest in this series is the early onset of panic attacks in those who develop any agoraphobic avoidance. Indeed, there seems to be a longer delay between onset of panic attacks and onset of agoraphobic avoidance in those who develop severe agoraphobia than in those who develop less severe phobic avoidance.

TABLE 3.1. *The ages of onset of panic attacks (First PA), panic disorder (PD), and agoraphobic avoidance (Avoidance) for 190 subjects according to panic disorder subtype*

	First PA	Age PD	Avoidance
Uncomplicated	30.1	31.7	–
Limited	27.5	29.8	30.4
Extensive	24.6	27.8	29.9

Overlapping diagnoses

Log–linear modelling techniques may be applied to categorical data to derive statistically significant interactions between the various categories.

The simplest model is chosen which is consistent with the data. Using the notation described by Feinberg (1977), the model derived from 190 panic disorder patients at initial interview is:

$$[SA] [SM] [CD] [MC] (\chi^2 = 50.5, df = 36, p > 0.05),$$

where S represents sex (male or female); A represents panic disorder subtype (uncomplicated, limited avoidance, or extensive avoidance); M represents simple phobia (present or absent); C represents social phobia (present or absent); and D represents depression (present or absent).

Thus, there is an interaction between the sex of the subject and both panic disorder subtype and simple phobia. Women report more agoraphobia and simple phobia than men. Also, social phobia is more frequent when either depression or simple phobia is present.

FOLLOW-UP STUDY

An attempt has been made to follow up the original series of patients with panic disorder and those with panic attacks who did not meet full criteria for the disorder. Some results are available on 96 subjects, 25 men and 71 women. At the follow-up interview, which on average was conducted about 4 years after initial contact, the SCID-UP was repeated for the intervening time period. The SCL-90, a patient self-report measure of 90 symptoms was also completed. The SCL-90 can be broken down into nine subscales covering anger and hostility, anxiety, depression, interpersonal sensitivity, obsessive–compulsive symptoms, paranoid ideation, phobic anxiety, psychotic symptoms, and somatization.

Of the 96 patients successfully followed-up, only 9 had either moved from the category of panic attacks without meeting full criteria into a panic disorder category, or developed worse agoraphobic avoidance. However, 26 had reduced agoraphobia, or no longer met criteria for panic disorder, or had fully recovered. Thus, 9 appeared worse, 26 improved, and 61 were unchanged. The SCL-90 scores, where available for both initial contact and follow-up, also indicate an improvement over the 4 years on *all* subscales. The largest changes are found in the subscales of anxiety, phobia, somatization, and depression, which were also the subscales scoring most highly at initial contact.

The overlap of diagnoses at follow-up was investigated by log–linear modelling, as described above. By comparing models at follow-up with models from the same population at initial interview, comments can be made on the course of the disorder. In the following models, social phobia is ignored since only 6 from 96 subjects were placed in this category. The initial model therefore differs from that previously described for the whole sample. The initial model is:

$$[M] [SA] [SD] (\chi^2 = 11.9, df = 15, p > 0.7),$$

where M represents Simple Phobia (present or absent); S represents sex (male or female); A represents panic disorder subtype (uncomplicated, limited avoidance or extensive avoidance); and D represents depression (present or absent). Here, there is no interaction between simple phobia and the other categories. Females report more phobic avoidance and depression than do men.

However, for these 96 subjects there is a change at follow-up, where, using the same categories, the derived model is:

$$[SA] [MA] [AD], (\chi^2 = 9.8, df = 12, p > 0.5).$$

Now, simple phobia and panic disorder subtype are interacting such that the presence of simple phobia is associated with increasing phobic avoidance, and phobic avoidance is also associated with the presence of depression. The interaction of sex and depression is no longer significant, but the association of female sex with increasing agoraphobia remains.

These models indicate the complexity of interactions in patients with panic disorder. It seems likely that simple phobias, where avoidance behaviour develops at an early age, predispose subjects who later panic to the problems of agoraphobia. Long-lasting agoraphobia, in both men and women, becomes associated with depression, overriding the initial predominance of female depressives.

SUBTYPES

Briggs (1989) has proposed that panic disorder should not merely be subtyped according to the degree of phobic avoidance present, but that account should be taken of the symptoms reported during panic attacks themselves. Using clustering techniques on a large sample of patients, he showed that patients could be placed in either of two groups, according to the prominence of respiratory symptoms during panic attacks. Patients with prominent respiratory symptoms responded better to imipramine, and reported more spontaneous panic attacks and perceived work impairment than did the group with more autonomic symptoms, which responded better to alprazolam and reported more situational panic attacks. This reported difference is now amenable to further investigation in future epidemiological studies where its significance can be assessed.

SUMMARY

Recent studies conducted by the University Department of Psychiatry in Leicester used operational criteria to investigate panic disorder. The concept of panic as a disorder rather than as a symptom is American, only recently gaining credence in Britain and Europe. Indeed, British psychiatrists have regarded panic disorder as a fiction, seeing panic as a response to the core symptom of agoraphobic avoidance behaviour. Ashcroft *et al.* (1987) noted that panic was a useful symptom complex but hesitated to embrace the disorder fully. Of necessity, studies of panic have had to utilize the American concept.

The Community Survey demonstrated the applicability of the concept of panic disorder in a British population, and the follow-up study should provide important information on the course of the disorder. Panic attacks have been shown to be common, and the similarity between subjects with infrequent panic attacks and those with panic disorder has led to refinements in diagnostic systems, now incorporated in DSM-III-R. The group of subjects with infrequent panic attacks may prove a fruitful area for aetiological research, perhaps representing a much purer form of panic disorder without the secondary complications of agoraphobia or depression.

Surprisingly, at follow-up the overall impression is of improvement. More subjects improved than worsened, and the notion that panic disorder patients use help-seeking behaviour and drain resources has in part been dispelled. Many subjects in the Community Survey did not want any intervention, and this was repeated at follow-up.

Information concerning age of onset and sex differences has been amassed. There is clearly a relationship between sex, depression, and agoraphobic avoidance. Women are over-represented in both categories, although with time men with avoidance become depressed as well. Early onset of panic attacks, or the presence of simple phobia are associated with later development of agoraphobia. Any comprehensive aetiological theory must account for these differences and also explain the responses of the subtypes with and without respiratory symptoms. It is hoped that the studies performed in Leicester have contributed to the understanding of panic and that the results will provide stimuli for further studies.

ACKNOWLEDGEMENTS

The above research studies were funded by Trent Regional Health Authority and UpJohn. We would also like to thank the staff and patients of the Uppingham Road Health Centre, Leicester for their help with the Community Survey and the Follow-Up Study, and Professor S. Brandon for his contributions and support.

REFERENCES

Agras, S., Sylvester, D., and Oliveau, D. (1969). The epidemiology of common fears and phobia. *Comprehensive Psychiatry*, **10**, 151–6.

APA (American Psychiatric Association) (1980). *Diagnostic and statistical manual of mental disorders* (3rd edn). APA, Washington DC.

APA (American Psychiatric Association) (1987). *Diagnostic and statistical manual of mental disorders* (3rd edn, revised). APA, Washington DC.

Angst, J. and Dobler-Mikola, A. (1985). The Zurich Study; V. Anxiety and phobia in young adults. *European Archives of Psychiatry and Neurological Sciences*, **235**, 171–8.

Ashcroft, G.W., Beaumont, G., Bonn, J., Brandon, S., Briggs, A., Clark, D., Davison, K., Gelder, M.G., Goldberg, D., and Herrington, R. (1987). Consensus statement on panic disorder. *British Journal of Psychiatry*, **150**, 557–8.

Brandon, S. (1989). Anxiety: does classification really help? In *Contempory themes in psychiatry* (eds K. Davison and A. Kerr). Gaskell, London.

Briggs, A.C. (1989). Subtyping panic disorder by symptom clusters. *Psychiatric Bulletin*, **13** (Abstr. Suppl. 2), 26.

Briggs, A.C. (1990). Panic: a follow-up study. *Psychiatric Bulletin*, **14** (Abstr. suppl. 3), 46.

Faravelli, C., Guerrini-Degl' Innocenti, B., and Giardinelli, L. (1989). Epidemiology of anxiety disorders in Florence. *Acta Pychiatrica Scandinavica*, **79**, 308–12.

Feinberg, S.T. (1977). *The analysis of cross-classified categorical data*. MIT Press, Cambridge, MA.

Klein, D.F. (1981). Anxiety reconceptualised. In *Anxiety — new research and changing concepts* (eds D.F. Klein and J.G. Rabkin). Raven Press, New York.

Marks, I. and Lader, M. (1973). Anxiety states (anxiety neurosis): A review. *Journal of Nervous and Mental Disease*, **156**, 3–18.

Regier, D.A., Myers, J.K., Kramer, M., Robins, L.N., Blazer, D.G., Hough, R.L., Eaton, W.W., and Locke, B.Z. (1984). The NIMH Epidemiologic Catchment Area Program historical context, major objectives, and study population characteristics. *Archives of General Psychiatry*, **41**, 934–41.

Spitzer, R.L. and Williams, J.B.W. (1983). *Structured clinical interview for DSM-III, Upjohn version*. Biometrics Research Department, New York State Psychiatric Institute.

Stirton, R.F. and Brandon, S. (1988). Preliminary report of a community survey of panic attacks and panic disorder. *Journal of the Royal Society of Medicine*, **81**, 392–3.

Surtees, P.G. and Sashidharan, S.P. (1986). Psychiatric morbidity in two matched community samples: a comparison of rates and risks in Edinburgh and St Louis. *Journal of Affective Disorders*, **10**, 101–13.

Uhlenhuth, E.H., Balter, M.B., Mellinger, G.D., Balter, M.B., Mellinger, G.D., Cisin, I.H., and Clinthorne, J. (1983). Symptom checklist syndromes in the general population. *Archives of General Psychiatry*, **40**, 1167–73.

Vollrath, M. and Angst, J. (1989). Outcome of panic and depression in a seven-year follow-up: results of the Zurich study. *Acta Psychiatrica Scandinavica*, **80**, 591–96.

von Korff, M.R., Eaton, W.W., and Keyl, P.M. (1985). The epidemiology of panic attacks and panic disorder: results of three community surveys. *American Journal of Epidemiology*, **122**, 970–81.

Weissman, M.M., Myers, J.K., and Harding, P.S. (1978). Psychiatric disorders in a U.S. urban community: 1975–1976. *American Journal of Psychiatry*, **135**, 459–62.

Weissman, M.M. (1990). Epidemiology of panic disorder and agoraphobia. *Psychiatric Medicine*, **8**, 3–13.

4

Symptomatology of panic disorder: an attempt to define the panic–agoraphobic spectrum phenomenology

G.B. CASSANO and M. SAVINO

INTRODUCTION

During the 1950s, Sir Martin Roth proposed the clinical entity 'panic attacks–agoraphobia'; this broke up the 'anxiety–depression continuum', and allowed clinicians and researchers to clearly separate the two categories. Roth (1959) also carried out a comparative clinical study outlining the wide symptomatological overlap between temporal lobe epilepsy and phobic–anxiety–derealization states.

Later on, Klein (1964) demonstrated the effectiveness of imipramine in patients with phobic-anxiety and a history of panic attacks. In 1967, Pitts and McClure (1967) induced panic attacks by sodium-lactate infusion in patients with panic disorder (PD) (APA 1987) and in predisposed subjects. More recently, Carr and Sheehan (1984) found Alprazolam to be effective in preventing lactate-induced panic attacks, while Liebowitz et al. (1984) and Sheehan et al. (1984) demonstrated the same property for imipramine and phenelzine. These observations provided both a 'pharmacological' and a 'biological dissection' for the wide area of 'neurotic' disorders; furthermore, a number of drugs capable of blocking and preventing panic attacks had become available.

The panic attack can be considered the main organizing principle in the area of neurotic disorders; it represents the core phenomenon possessing fundamental diagnostic value for PD. Often, however, panic attack symptoms are less clear and distinct than in the classic clinical descriptions, and associated features as well as the consequences of panic attacks may mask the core phenomena. This usually happens when PD is attenuated or has an early onset, or when it is followed by mood disorders that may be prevalent in the patient's experience.

The term '*panic–agoraphobic spectrum*' includes the whole range of possible manifestations, subjective experiences and consequences of panic phenomena, which are not always recognized and whose psychopathological, diagnostic, and therapeutic significance is often underestimated.

The concept of a 'panic–agoraphobic spectrum' should allow the psychiatrist to detect a panic attack even if it is atypical and/or remote in the patient's and in the family's history, and to reconstruct the various steps in the evolution of the disorder up to its definitive appearance. Moreover, the analytical detection and assessment of panic–agoraphobic spectrum phenomena enable the clinician to consider the frequent co-occurrence of PD with other psychopathological features (Cassano *et al.* 1991), such as bipolar and other disorders — obsessive–compulsive (OCD), and eating disorders — even if the typical panic attack is not sharply evident in the clinical picture. The precise recognition of co-morbidity phenomena in the area of 'neurotic' and personality disorders permits a better classification and a targeted treatment of anxiety and mood disorders.

The associated features and co-morbid disorders that are frequently observed in patients with PD are shown in Fig. 4.1, according to our data derived from a study on 302 PD patients (Cassano *et al.* 1990).

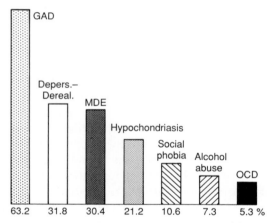

FIG. 4.1. Concomitant features in 302 PD patients.

PANIC ATTACKS AND ANTICIPATORY ANXIETY

Panic attack is a sudden experience of distress, catastrophic menace and intense suffering accompanied by severe neurovegetative symptoms, respiratory and cardiovascular phenomena — such as dyspnea and tachicardia — and neurological symptoms — such as tremor and dizziness.

These phenomena are commonly followed by the fear of a heart attack, and of losing control or going crazy. Derealization–depersonalization symptoms are present in about 30 per cent of all cases (Cassano *et al.* 1989). In some cases, the fear of dying or going crazy may not be present and the patient may ask for cardiological, neurological or otorhinolaryngological consultations, showing little apprehension and anxiety.

Panic attacks — the organizing principle in the diagnosis of PD — also play a pivotal role as outcome measures of the pharmacological treatment. They disappear after a pharmacological block, leading in most cases to the resolution of anticipatory anxiety, phobias and avoidant behaviour.

After both situational and unexpected panic attacks, a complex symptomatology may appear. The latter aspect, which sometimes obscures nuclear anxious spells, is represented by the anticipatory anxiety, the fear of being trapped, the avoidant behaviour, and the need for an accompanying companion and medical help.

The sudden-onset, uncontrollable, short-lived, often unexpected panic attack differs from *anticipatory anxiety*, which is due to the expectation of subsequent attacks, and to the fear of situations specifically related to them. Anticipatory anxiety can be largely controlled and managed by the patient who must, however, be taught to recognize the two different anxious phenomena.

Anticipatory anxiety tends to lower the panic threshold and favours the onset of behavioural and neurovegetative symptoms such as hyperventilation, which can trigger an attack.

Secondary hypochondriasis may derive from major panic attacks, as well as from minor panic attacks, which are often obscured by it. The *hypochondriac thinking* is often focused on the fear of having a cardiovascular disease, or a respiratory or neurological illness. A *secondary simple phobia* may be determined by conditioning associations with panic attacks. *Secondary social phobia* is often reported by panic patients, and is linked to the fear of having a panic attack, losing control, or doing something that will embarrass or puzzle bystanders. Such worries may produce severe avoidant behaviour of social situations (Perugi *et al.* 1990).

There may be an associated state of *secondary demoralization*, characterized by anxious–dysphoric mood (Fig. 4.2).

The proposed descriptive approach, which has been widely adopted in the area of 'neurotic-anxious' disorders, is reminiscent of the psychiatry of the late 1800s, as recorded in the contributions of the French authors of the 'ictus bulbaire', the 'angoisse bulbaire', and the 'ictus emotif' (Brissand 1890); it also appears to be close to Lopez-Ibor's (1950) description of 'anxious thymopathy' or 'endothymic anxiety', a condition considered as 'not neurotic, not reactive', but due to an 'endothymic' factor.

The concept of a 'panic–agoraphobic spectrum' should help the clini-

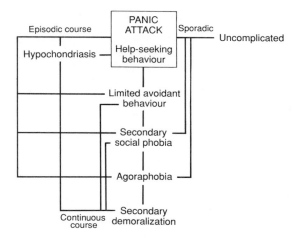

FIG. 4.2. Evolution of PD.

cian to detect the panic attack even if it occurs in an atypical, incomplete or hidden way.

The panic–agoraphobic spectrum comprises all of the following: (a) *panic attacks*, (b) *anxious expectation*, (c) *polyphobic features*, (d) *avoidant behaviour*, (e) *reassurance sensitivity*, (f) *help-seeking behaviour*, (g) *maladaptive behaviour*, (h) *predisposing and prodromal factors*, (i) *physiological sensitivity to some substances* (Table 4.1). In the different phases of the course of the disorder one aspect may prevail over the others, so producing a high degree of variability in the symptomatological and behavioural patterns; in some subjects such patterns can simulate other clinical entities.

TABLE 4.1. *Panic–agoraphobic spectrum*

A — Panic attacks
B — Anxious expectation
C — Polyphobias
D — Avoidance
E — Reassurance sensitivity
F — Help-seeking behaviour
G — Maladaptive behaviour
H — Predisposing or prodromal factors
I — Physiological sensitivity to substances

A — Panic attacks, post- and inter-critical phenomena

A typical *panic attack* — whether unexpected or situational, spontaneous or drug-induced (i.e. by caffeine, cocaine, LSD) — is easy to recognize, and may follow one of various patterns (Table 4.2): many attacks every day, a few attacks per month, or periodic 'clusters' of attacks. A panic attack can be an isolated event in the patient's lifespan, or, more rarely, an almost continuous phenomenon, describable as 'panic status'. Typical panic attacks are sometimes replaced by minor atypical ones, with isolated respiratory, cardiac, intestinal, or neurological symptoms. The clinical picture is nevertheless completed by a sense of an overwhelming threat, sometimes by an intense fear of dying, losing control, or going crazy. Minor attacks may be associated with some respiratory symptoms, such as the sudden feeling of a difficulty in deep breathing. In these cases the hypochondriac worry of having a respiratory illness, or the fear of something that is blocking breathing function, may mask the critical panic event. The fear of losing control over the anus or bladder sphincters can be found in other patients, who are therefore avoiding places that don't have a toilet immediately available. Various *somatic areas* can be affected by critical panic spells: feelings of sudden paralysis, a block while walking, a loss of balance, and an overwhelming collapse, are all quite frequent.

On the *psychological side*, an attack may merely take the form of a fear of losing control over impulses involving auto- and hetero-aggressivity, as when a patient is disturbed by open windows, isolated places, knives and guns.

The *post-critical and inter-critical symptomatology* is closely related to panic spells and has a special clinical relevance. A sense of numbness, tiredness or nausea, a headache, hypersensitivity to noises, light and heat, depression, depersonalization–derealization and other misperceptions, a

TABLE 4.2. *A — Critical, post-critical, and inter-critical phenomena*

Major panic attack	Unexpected	Sporadic-isolated
	Situational	Recurrent-episodic
		High frequency-continuous 'panic state'
	Spontaneous	
	Drug-induced	

With or without help-seeking behaviour

Minor panic attack
Atypical panic attack
Post-critical and inter-critical symptomatology

TABLE 4.3. *Clinical features of PD patients with and without derealization and depersonalization (DD)*

	PD + DD (*n* = 104) 34.8% *M*	PD (*n* = 195) 65.2% *M*	*p*
Age	33.7	38.9	0.001
Age at onset	26.1	30.3	0.001
Phobia scale factors			
Agoraphobia	5.0	4.0	0.004
Hypochondriasis	4.5	3.5	0.01
Global judgement	6.0	5.3	0.04

sense of unstable balance or of 'walking on rubber', are all possible sequels to panic attacks, and may persist for days or even months. Such interval phenomena make a substantial contribution to the development and maintenance of phobic avoidance.

Derealization–depersonalization (DD) is quite frequent in people having PD. In our clinical samples we found DD symptoms present in nearly 35 per cent of PD patients (Cassano *et al.* 1989) (Table 4.3), and these showed an earlier age at onset, more severe agoraphobia and hypochondriasis, and a poorer global judgement in the phobia scale factors.

Panic patients may experience a sensation of inner division as a primary event; they may see themselves as a robot, an automaton, or as in a movie.

In others the attack is followed by severe depression with a sudden onset, which continues in the inter-critical phase (Cassano *et al.* 1989); in most such cases panic attacks are overlooked by clinicians who overrate the mood disorder.

Within the large group of patients who ask for help because of an anxious symptomatology, many do so because of atypical minor attacks, or because of post-critical and inter-critical phenomena in the absence of clear-cut major panic attacks.

Panic attacks may be accompanied by different feelings and expressed in radically different emotional styles — from the tragic–dramatic to the histrionic–manipulative — with a sense of sudden death or a sense of public embarrassment and humiliation; both temperamental and cultural aspects contribute to a kaleidoscopic phenomenology. In a considerable number of subjects it is experienced without anxiety and fear and with a predominant experience of anger.

These critical manifestations favour the development and maintenance of phobic ideation and avoidant behaviour; they fuel and aggravate anticipatory anxiety and produce a severe disability.

B — Anxious expectation

Freud (1895) accurately described *anxious expectation*, which is frequent in these patients and has great diagnostic relevance. The fear of having the next panic attack, with its catastrophic experience of terror — 'phobophobia' — is linked with 'anticipatory anxiety' and with the 'persistent alarm state' (Table 4.4), both of which are key features of anxious expectation. Anxious expectation, as critical and post-critical symptomatology, induces, blow-up and maintains phobic–avoidant behaviour patterns.

TABLE 4.4. *B — Anxious expectation*

Anticipatory anxiety	Preceding exposure to phobic stimuli	Claustro-agoraphobia Polyphobias Secondary social phobia
	Risk of having panic attacks	Phobophobia
Persistent alarm state	Fear of suffocation or of having a heart attack	Sudden death phobia
	Fear of losing control or going crazy	Mental illness phobia

Anticipatory anxiety mainly regards specific areas, phobic objects and situations, such as closed and/or open places, and crowded places; the real possibility — or a fantasy — of a confrontation with them may enhance this type of anxiety and lower the threshold of panic attacks.

A *persistent alarm state* is a general condition of alertness and great insecurity, deriving from the risk of having a new major or minor panic attack; it is linked with a constant, overwhelming threat of a mental or physical breakdown — such as an anticipated severe physical illness, a respiratory choke, a stroke, a heart attack, or sudden insanity.

While a patient may be able to partly master anticipatory anxiety, which is linked with specific phobic situations, he will not be able to control the persistent alarm state, which is related to the fear of a sudden loss of his physical or mental health. When such a distressing and persistent condition affects the whole life-style of a patient, it may be difficult to detect some of the less typical core phenomena of PD. These patients seem to live in a seismic area troubled by frequent major or minor earthquakes, and their anxious expectation is linked with a deep, extreme sense of instability.

Among patients suffering from PD, a considerable number show anticipatory anxiety phases over a persistent alarm state. In these patients a panic attack may easily be overlooked and misdiagnosed; whereas a targeted interview would reveal the fear of being exposed to the typical phobic stimuli, the fear of having a heart attack or losing control and being humiliated.

C — Polyphobias

Phobic phenomena (Table 4.5) may be largely grouped in the 'claustro-agoraphobic' condition. Most PD patients are very sensitive to open and/ or closed spaces, and to stale air and temperature changes — they often say: 'I like the winter . . . In a room, I have to switch off the heating and open the windows.' When the temperature or the CO_2 rate increases, these patients may start panicking; one hypothesis put forward to account for this has been that of a chemoreceptor dysregulation (Liebowitz *et al.* 1984), probably determining a hypersensitivity to warm and stale air, and ultimately to closed spaces.

TABLE 4.5. *C — Polyphobias*

Claustro-agoraphobia
Secondary social phobia
Pathophobia and secondary hypochondriasis
Drug phobia
Secondary simple phobias (due to conditioning associations)

Other polyphobic features, if accurately explored, are very valuable in diagnosing less typical cases of PD; the specific life-style of many PD patients may be affected by these phenomena, both at the cognitive and the behavioural levels. Even so, avoidant, passive and dependent aspects of these patients' personalities, often disappear after a specific anti-panic drug treatment.

Special attention must be devoted to the phobic avoidance of social situations secondary to the fear of having a panic attack. Patients afraid of being embarrassed in public, or of being humiliated by the physical or psychological symptoms of an attack while they are performing, may show a cognitive and behavioural pattern that is indistinguishable from that of primary social-phobics. A 'secondary social phobia' (Perugi *et al.* 1990) is, in fact, a frequent occurrence in the PD population, and should be accurately detected and differentiated from primary social phobia, both for diagnostic and for therapeutic purposes. Primary social phobia responds

TABLE 4.6a. *Primary and secondary social phobia*

	Primary social phobia (n = 25) $\bar{X}$	Secondary social phobia (n = 26) $\bar{X}$	Panic disorder agoraphobia (n = 82) $\bar{X}$	p Scheffé	
Index age	30.9	34.7	41.0	0.001	P < A
Age at onset	17.0 P < A, S	27.1	28.4	0.001	
Family history					
Social phobia	4.0	0.0	2.4	ns	
Panic disorder	4.0	30.8	19.5	< 0.05	
Major depression	40.0	26.9	25.6	ns	

TABLE 4.6b. *Primary and secondary social phobia*

Concomitant disorders

	Primary social phobia (n = 25)		Secondary social phobia (n = 26)		Panic disorder agoraphobia (n = 82)		
	n	%	n	%	n	%	p
Generalized anxiety	9	36.0	12	46.2	32	39.0	ns
Alcohol abuse	5	20.0	2	7.7	5	6.1	ns
Drug abuse	1	4.0	2	7.7	5	6.1	ns
Obsessive compulsive	0	0.0	5	19.2	2	2.4	< 0.001
Major depression	9	36.0	11	42.3	22	26.8	ns
School phobia	7	28.0	8	30.8	22	26.8	ns

P = Primary social phobia, S = Secondary social phobia, A = Agoraphobia with panic attacks.

specifically to phenelzine (Leibowitz *et al.* 1985) and to fluoxetine (Deltito *et al.* 1990). In our studies comparing social phobia with PD and PD plus secondary social phobia (Table 4.6a, b), we found an earlier age at onset in patients with primary social phobia and a longer duration of the illness in this group. Patients with PD and secondary social phobia showed a higher family loading for PD than patients suffering from primary social phobia and those with PD. As far as concomitant disorders are concerned, OCD was significantly more common in patients with panic attacks and secondary social phobia.

The pathophobic aspects that can produce a '*secondary hypochondriac syndrome*' in many PD patients, focus mainly on the fear of respiratory, cardiological, neurological or mental illnesses. This clinical condition is often linked with a remote panic attack and/or with mild but persistent post-critical symptoms, i.e. fear of a severe respiratory dysfunction in patients with dyspnea, fear of a brain tumour in patients with a long-standing sense of instability in walking, and fear of heart disease in patients with frequent tachicardia. In these cases, an evaluation of age at onset, family history, course, history of panic attacks, and response to specific treatment (Cassano *et al.* 1985) allow the clinician to distinguish primary from secondary hypochondriasis. In many cases, panic attacks may be triggered by the sudden news of the heart attack of a colleague or friend, or simply the sudden death of an unknown person. Knowledge of a severe disease that has anticipated the loss of, or separation from, a loved person may also be connected with the onset of the disorder. Thus, the hypochondriac alarm state is mixed with separation anxiety feelings.

The fear of mental illnesses, of 'going crazy', is clinically relevant and important from a diagnostic point of view. It is accompanied by intense anxiety and is often expressed in an obsessive way. Some PD patients, among those with psychiatric disorders, are probably the only ones to express a fear of going mad. The phobic condition is that of a major mental illness, such as 'schizophrenia'. In this particular group of individuals, symptoms of derealization–depersonalization and, more rarely, impulse dyscontrol are often associated with, or follow, panic attacks.

'Drug-phobia' is also common in PD patients; it affects their compliance with treatments and is often reinforced by hypersensitivity to some substances, including trycyclic antidepressants (TCA), which makes the management of these patients more complicated. Most of these patients tell us '. . . I am idiosyncratic, and allergic to all drugs.' They attentively read the explanatory leaflet, and refuse to take the drug because they are scared by its possible cardio-vascular toxicity. In these cases admission to hospital is often a precondition for pharmacological therapy.

Less typical phobias are also frequent in subjects with PD. When the panic spells are rare and mild, secondary phobias due to conditioning associations — such as the fear of sexual activity, or of eating, secondary social phobia, secondary hypochondriasis or pathophobia — may lead the clinician to give inappropiate diagnoses, such as sexual disorder, specific phobia, anorexia nervosa, social phobia, hypochondriasis, and depression.

D — Avoidant behaviour

In about 20 per cent of subjects with PD it is not easy to identify a clear *avoidant behaviour* (Cassano *et al.* 1985). Though a number of these patients feel independent and able to go everywhere, some of them admit that they often need to 'force themselves'. This kind of statement may suggest that the clinician should examine the symptomatology of the panic–agoraphobic spectrum.

Avoidant behaviour (Table 4.7) and/or a strict dependency on an accompanying companion, may be the only evident consequence of panic attacks occurring in the past history of some patients. In these cases the main avoidant symptoms of the panic–agoraphobic spectrum are linked to the fear of being alone, or to worries about losing the accompanying companion or the way back.

The widespread avoidance of close, crowded, or open spaces, where it may be hard to escape or be helped by others, and a vague sense of being trapped, associated with various conditions, may induce a large spectrum of forms of avoidant behaviour.

TABLE 4.7. *D — Avoidant Behaviour (or forced self-exposure)*

Being alone at home or outside	
Travelling alone	
Open and/or closed places	
Public performances	Speeches
	Lectures
	Lessons
	Meetings
Other places, situations	Hospitals and medical services
	Dentist
	Queueing
	Eating
	Sexual activity
	Clothes, ties, rings,
	Plaster casts
	Seat belts

Phobic avoidance often interferes with a subject's social relationships; a patient may be afraid to speak in front of more than one person, or avoid restaurants, cafés, post offices and banks. Some patients are afraid of queueing because of their fear of falling down. Others do not use objects that may give a sense of claustrophobia, such as seat belts, rings, high-necked shirts, and tight clothes. Some ask for certificates allowing them not to use a safety belt in a car or plane; others cut their clothes to make their chest and abdominal respiratory activity easier. Thus, there is a large number of forms of avoidant behaviour that can prevail over the other characteristics of the PD. When the attack is not easy to recognize or recall, the clinician should be able to recognize panic patients because of their avoidance of the dentist, hospitals, and objects or situations involving the medical area. If there is no clear avoidance conduct, a detailed interview may reveal that the patient makes indeed a forced self-exposure, with different degrees of distress.

The inability to stay alone at home, or do things in public such as giving lectures or lessons, receiving dental treatment or wearing ties, belts, tight clothes, or rings, may prove to be the most disturbing and disabling major aspects of an underlying PD. A wide and heterogeneous spectrum of avoidance behaviour may take up the foreground, compared with other features of the disorder. Thus, besides all types of avoidant behaviour, a previous history of panic attacks should be enquired into.

E — Reassurance sensitivity

A typical feature of PD patients is their extreme *reassurance sensitivity* (Table 4.8). This producing histrionic, demanding traits in these subjects, who can easily be reassured and encouraged. Their high degree of responsiveness to any kind of suggestive stimuli had led to their being considered inauthentic, and they have often been given the pejorative labels of 'neurotics' and 'hysterics'.

Reassurance sensitivity favours attachment to a significant friend or

TABLE 4.8. *E — Reassurance sensitivity*

Reduction of anxiety through:		
'Protective' objects	BZs	Umbrella
	Drinks	Sun-glasses
	Sweets	Bicycle
	Cane	Trolley
	Hat	
Accompanying companion	Spouse	
	Family member	
	Friend	
	Doctor	
Safety measures	Sitting near the exit	
	Available telephone	
	Available medical services	
	'Ship setting sail'	
Magic rituals		
Superstitious practices		

relative; it can also produce a kind of behaviour close to 'magic and superstitious thinking'. These patients take protective objects with them; they may keep BZs (benzodiazepines) or antiarrythmic drugs in their pockets; others are incapable of travelling by plane, train, or car without a bottle of water; others may use walking-sticks, or go out with a dog or an accompanying companion. They adopt 'safety measures' in terms of checking out any available emergency room or any way of escape. If they must go out alone, they often go through strict rituals in preparing for a departure, even before short trips; they take complicated precautions to avoid any possible risk of anxiety, and they tell someone in whom they have absolute trust. We have called this behavioural pattern 'ship setting sail'.

The marked tendency to become attached to significant others is associated with dependency on any person, object, or situation capable of reassuring them and alleviating their anxiety. The bizarre bond that links these patients with umbrellas, canes, or dark glasses, or with an 'accompanying companion', may induce the psychiatrist to make an incorrect diagnosis of personality disorder, especially if their inexplicable dependence on protective objects predominates over other forms of behaviour. In the same way some of the 'safety measures' chosen by PD patients, such as their habit of sitting near the exit in cinemas and theatres, and their preference for living near medical care centres, may be overlooked. Rituals, magic thinking, and superstitious behaviour patterns may be quite common, and they may lead some PD patients to be misdiagnosed as people suffering from OCD or schizotypal personality disorder.

F — Help-seeking behaviour

One characteristic of some particular phases of the evolution of PD is the continuous help-seeking behaviour that springs from reassurance sensitivity; especially in the early phases of the disorder, this mechanism tends to promote a dependency on 'protective' persons, objects, and situations. The main trait in the personality of some patients may be their continuous search for help, together with their sensitivity to reassurance.

Typical *help-seeking behaviour* (Table 4.9) involves family members, friends, and physicians; if successful it progressively reinforces dependency.

It is easy to find these patients in emergency units and medical care centres; some of them may even sleep in a car parked close to the hospital.

A major characteristic of some of these subjects is their great interest in everything involving the health and medical area — doctors, illnesses, and death. PD patients often ask for repeated medical examinations and lab

TABLE 4.9. *F — Help-seeking behaviour*

Family members
Friends
Doctors
Laboratory tests
Emergency medical services
Hospital admission

tests or other diagnostic procedures. They may be admitted several times to hospitals, where they may, over prolonged periods, receive incorrect pharmacological or inappropriate psychotherapeutic treatments that favour a chronic evolution of the disorder. In some cases hospitals, doctors, psychotherapists, and sedative drug dependence may become the predominant features.

Though PD patients may sometimes avoid the clinician because of his drugs, in most of them the doctor plays a great reassuring role and is often needed as a saviour; thus, the relationships between a PD patient and his or her clinician is very different from that of patients suffering from primary hypochondriasis.

G — Maladaptive behaviour

Like other chronic disabling disorders, PD may produce personality changes and forms of *maladaptive behaviour* (Table 4.10) severe enough to mask the most typical manifestations of the disorder. Many patients cut down their work load or stop working altogether, and limit their social and leisure activities. They lead a restricted life governed by refusal and self-prohibition, and dominated by fears, constrictions and forms of avoidant behaviour; they also impose it on their partner and their siblings. Self-denial and self-imposed limitations in a variety of areas characterize these subjects' lives and often appear as the predominant aspect of the disorder, leading either to an attitude of anger and rebellion, or to passiveness and victimism. Drug and alcohol abuse may be a frequent and serious complication of the disorder.

TABLE 4.10. *G — Maladaptive behaviour*

Chronic disabling disorder	Family
Reassurance and dependency	Work
Attachment and 'histrionic style'	Leisure time and social interactions
Secondary demoralization	Substance abuse

These patients' attitudes towards others may become 'histrionic' and manipulative; their reactions to separation may appear to be dramatic, and their attachment to others theatrical and exaggerated. They may change their married relationships or look for sexual partners exclusively on the basis of their reassuring qualities. Thus, a young woman may choose, or stay with, an old or impotent husband because she believes he will never get tired of her or leave her in dangerous situations.

If there are no secondary maladaptive features, the romantic life and sexual activity of PD subjects are normal. So long as they feel safe at home and elsewhere, these patients can have normal work, leisure, and sexual activity. In these respects PD clearly differs even from mild depression, which produces severe sexual, work and leisure impairment (Cassano *et al.* 1983).

H — Physiological sensitivity to substances

A *low threshold to physical and chemical stimuli*, as well as to life events, may characterize patients with disorders belonging to panic–agoraphobic spectrum. Caffeine, cocaine, amphetamine, or marijuana (Table 4.11) may trigger the first panic attack, which then determines the subsequent complex development of the disorder. Similarly, various stressors may determine the first, as well as subsequent, attacks. PD often starts after a period of stress-inducing conditions, such as excessive work commitments, or the use of stimulating drugs. A substantial decrease in sleeping time, or a prolonged period of tension and worry due to life events may also lead up to it.

TABLE 4.11. *H — Physiological sensitivity*

Hypersensitivity to	Caffeine
	Cannabis
	Amphetamine
	Cocaine
	Thyroxine
	TCA (?)

Some patients report typical conditions of hyperstimulation, with anxiety and agitation, with or without panic attacks, during BZ withdrawal or after the administration of TCAs. In depressive patients this kind of reaction should allow the clinician to infer a possible co-morbidity with PD, or a concomitant attenuated form of the panic–agoraphobic spectrum, as when an anxious patient refuses TCAs because of a belief that he is 'allergic' to them and other kinds of drugs.

I — Predisposing or prodromal

Mitral valve prolapse, separation anxiety in childhood and school phobia, are common *predisposing or prodromal factors* to PD (Table 4.12). Prodromal and predisposing factors may have a predictive value when they are observed early in the siblings of patients with PD.

TABLE 4.12. *I — Predisposing or prodromal*

Separation anxiety disorder in childhood
School phobia
Mitral valve prolapse

We have observed cases of PD appearing together with school phobia or separation anxiety in infancy (Perugi *et al*. 1988).

Separation anxiety and school phobia in childhood have an important diagnostic and prognostic value. They point to a more severe disorder, an earlier onset, a heavier family loading, and a greater risk of developing avoidant behaviour.

In our clinical samples of PD patients, with and without a history of separation anxiety in childhood (Table 4.13), the first group showed a significantly lower age at onset of PD, and an earlier onset of avoidant behaviour than the second group.

TABLE 4.13. *Panic disorder with and without previous separation anxiety*

	PD (No. 200) M	PD+SA (No. 64) M	*p*
Percentage of the total PD sample	75.8	24.2	
Age at onset of PD	28.7	25.4	0.008
Age at onset of avoidant behaviour	31.1	26.3	0.001
Avoidant behaviour (global impression)	5.5	6.0	ns

'PURE' PD AND 'PD SPECTRUM'

Though panic attacks represent the nuclear aspect of PD, patients showing atypical disorders in terms of symptomatology and course are quite frequent in clinical practice. Patients with PD often show symptoms of generalized anxiety, depression, and obsessions (Sheehan *et al*. 1980), and

TABLE 4.14. *Demographic data, diagnoses and co-morbid disorders in PD patients*

	PD-spectrum (150)		Pure PD (90)	
	M	*s*	*M*	*s*
Age	38.4	11.7	31.4	9.3 **
Age at onset:				
First panic attack	28.7	10.4	26.7	8.7
Avoidant behaviour	31.4	11.2	27.0	8.1 *
Length of illness	9.7	11.2	4.7	5.5 **
Gender		%		%
Females		60.0		58.9
Diagnoses				
PD		27.3		33.3
Limited phobic avoidance		18.0		17.8
Extensive phobic avoidance		54.7		48.9
Co-morbid disorders				
Depersonalization/derealization		34.7		30.0
Alcohol abuse		5.3		–
BZs abuse		7.3		–
OCD		5.3		–
MDE		30.7		7.8 **
Social phobia		10.7		7.8
Separation anxiety and school phobia		26.0		22.2

* $p < 0.05$, ** $p < 0.01$.

the use of hierarchical models may impair a comprehensive diagnostic assessment. With the aim of exploring the symptomatological and course characteristics of different forms of PD, we have studied the clinical features of two groups of PD patients. One group, comprising 150 patients, was selected on the basis of broad, hierarchy-free criteria (PD spectrum); the second group was made up of the first 90 patients recruited for the 'World-wide Upjohn Study for Panic Disorder' (Klerman *et al.* 1986). These were chosen on the basis of restrictive criteria, i.e. patients had had at least one panic attack every week in the last month, without co-morbid disorders.

The comparison of these two groups of PD patients showed that demographic, clinical, and symptomatological features were similar in the two groups (Tables 4.14–15). The higher age at onset of PD and of avoidant behaviour in the PD-spectrum group could be accounted for by the inclusion criteria used for the pure-PD group, which required a relatively

TABLE 4.15. *Symptomatological features of PD patients*

	PD-Spectrum (150)		Pure PD (90)	
	M	s	M	s
Major panic attacks				
Unexpected	7.2	11.3	11.6	15.7*
Situational	3.9	8.3	5.9	14.0
Minor panic attacks				
Unexpected	9.9	15.0	30.5	60.2**
Situational	7.0	10.7	13.8	27.6*
Anticipatory anxiety (%)	50.2	29.8	59.4	55.0
Avoidant behaviour	5.8	3.1	5.3	3.5
Total Ham-D	11.0	4.0	10.4	4.4
HSCL-90				
Anxiety	2.03	0.8	1.90	0.8
Phobic anxiety	1.93	1.1	1.78	1.1
Somatization	1.69	0.8	1.69	0.8
Depression	1.54	0.7	1.40	0.7
Obsession-Compulsion	1.51	0.8	1.33	0.9*
Sensitivity	1.18	0.8	1.11	0.8
Hostility–anger	1.04	0.8	1.06	0.9
Paranoidism	0.99	0.7	0.98	0.8
Psychoticism	0.98	0.6	0.98	0.7

* $p < 0.05$, ** $p < 0.01$.

high frequency of attacks. The demographic and clinical data demonstrated that the entire panic–agoraphobic spectrum covers and unifies the various clinical manifestations of a multi-faced single disorder.

CONCLUDING REMARKS

The concept of a 'panic–agoraphobic spectrum', and the supersession of a hierarchical approach which excluded a diagnosis of PD in the presence of 'more pervasive' concomitant disorders, are factors that widen the boundaries in the area of panic manifestations. Even if atypical and less severe forms of panic were included within the 'panic-disorder spectrum', in our clinical sample, that entity seems to maintain the characteristics — in terms of course and treatment response — that have conferred on PD its central position within the anxiety disorders.

An accurate detection of typical PD symptoms, among the ill-defined area of 'neurotic disorders', allows clinicians to isolate a discrete psychopathological entity, which responds to specific drug treatments. The detailed description of the less typical features and lesser-known phenomena of PD aims to offer a comprehensive picture of the 'panic–agoraphobic spectrum' that is clinically meaningful, and to offer a significant advance in research.

This approach permits a clearer identification of lifespan and intra-episodic co-morbidity, as many patients with mood disorders, OCD, somatoform, eating, and personality disorders may show incomplete signs and attenuated symptoms belonging to less typical forms in the panic–agoraphobic spectrum.

As the less typical forms of this disorder, as of others, are by far the most common, the proposed analytical exploration and systematic evaluation of PD symptom patterns should have a significant didactic and practical impact.

REFERENCES

APA (American Psychiatric Association) / Committee on Nomenclature and Statistics (1987). *Diagnostic and statistical manual of mental disorders*, (3rd edn revised) The American Psychiatric Association Washington, DC.

Brissaud, M. (1890). De l'anxieté paroxystique. *Semaine Médicale*, 410–11.

Carr, D.B. and Sheehan, D.V. (1984). Panic anxiety. A new biological model. *Journal of Clinical Psychiatry*, **145**, 323–30.

Cassano, G.B., Maggini, C., and Akiskal, H.S. (1983). Short term, subchronic and chronic sequelae of affective disorders. *Psychiatric Clinics of North America*, **6**, 55.

Cassano, G.B., Deltito, J., Perugi, G., Mauri, M., and Petracca, A. (1985). Il disturbo da attacchi di panico e agorafobia. *Quaderni Italiani di Psichiatria*, **IV**, 1, 41–74.

Cassano, G.B., Petracca, A., Perugi, G., Toni, C., Tundo, A., and Roth, M. (1989*a*). Derealization and panic attacks: a clinical evaluation on 150 patients with panic disorder/agoraphobia. *Comprehensive Psychiatry*, **30**, 1, 5–12.

Cassano, G.B., Musetti, L., Perugi, G., and Akiskal, H.S. (1989*b*). The nature of depression presenting concomitantly with panic disorder. *Comprehensive Psychiatry*, **30** (6), 1–10.

Cassano, G.B., Perugi, G., and Musetti L. (1990). Co-morbidity in panic disorder. *Psychiatric Annals*, **20**, 517–21.

Cassano, G.B., Savino, M., Musetti, L., and Perugi, G. (1991). In *Co-morbidity between mood and anxiety disorders*. Proceedings of the international meeting Serotonin-Related Psychiatric Syndromes: Clinical and Therapeutic Links, Venice, 29–31 March 1990. Royal Society of Medicine Services, 165, London, New York.

Deltito, J.A., Poeschla, B.D., Stam, M., and Martin, Y. (1991). In *Monoamine oxidase inhibitors or fluoxetine in the treatment of avoidant personality disorder*. Proceedings of the international meeting Serotonin-Related Psychiatric

Syndromes: Clinical and Therapeutic Links, Venice, 29–31 March 1990. Royal Society of Medicine Services, 165, London, New York.

Freud, S. (1895). On the grounds for detaching a particular syndrome from neuroasthenia under the description 'anxiety neurosis'. In *the standard edition of the complete psychological works of Sigmund Freud*, Hogarth Press, London, Vol. 7, (ed. J. Strachey). 1961.

Klein, D.F. (1964). Delineation of two drug-responsive anxiety syndromes. *Psychopharmacologia*, **5**, 397–408.

Klerman, G.L., Coleman, J.H., and Purpura, R.P. (1986). The design and conduct of the Upjohn Cross-National Collaborative Panic Study. *Psychopharmacological Bulletin*, **22** (1), 59–64.

Liebowitz, M.R., Fyer, A.J., Gorman, J.M., Dillon, D., Appleby, I.L., Levy, J. *et al.* (1984). Lactate provocation of panic attacks-I. Clinical and behavioral findings. *Archives of General Psychiatry*, **41**, 764–70.

Liebowitz, M.R., Gorman, J.M., Fyer, A.J., Campeas, R., Levin, A., Davies. S., and Klein, D.F. (1985). Psychopharmacological treatment of social phobia. *Psychopharmacological Bulletin*, **21**, 610–14.

Lopez-Ibor, J.P. (1950). Angoisse, existence, vitalité. *Evolution Psychiatrique*, **2**, 263–93.

Perugi, G., Deltito, J., Soriani, A., Musetti, L., Petracca, A., Nisita, C. *et al.* (1988). Relationships between panic disorder and separation anxiety with school phobia. *Comprehensive Psychiatry*, **29**, 98–107.

Perugi, G., Simonini, E., Savino, M., Mengali, F., Cassano, G.B., and Akiskal, H.S. (1990). Primary and secondary social phobia: psychopathologic and familial differentiations. *Comprehensive Psychiatry*, **31**, 3, 245–52.

Pitts, F.N. and McClure, J.N. (1967). Lactate metabolism in anxiety neurosis. *New England Journal of Medicine*, **277**, 1329–36.

Roth, M. (1959). The phobic Anxiety-depersonalization syndrome. *Proceedings of the Royal Society of Medicine*, 587–95.

Sheehan, D.V., Ballenger, J., and Jacobsen, G. (1980). Treatment of endogenous anxiety with phobic, hysterical, and hypochondriacal symptoms. *Archives of General Psychiatry*, **37**, 51–9.

Sheehan, D.V., Cleycomb, J.B., and Surman, O.S. (1984). In *The relative efficacy of alprazolam phenelzine and imipramine in treating panic attacks and phobias*, American Psychiatric Association (ed.), Abstracts of the Scientific Proceedings of the 137th Annual Meeting of the American Pychiatric Association, Los Angeles.

5

Growth hormone stimulation by clonidine in panic disorder

BERNARD J. CARROLL

INTRODUCTION

A theme mentioned by Dr Leonard (Chapter 10) and repeated in several other chapters of this volume, is that there may be some overlap of the neurobiology of panic disorders and depressive disorders. Because of the long history of neuroendocrine studies in depression, it is not surprising that similar exploratory studies have been conducted in panic disorders. The rationale for neuroendocrine studies in psychiatric conditions is by now well known: evidence of dysregulated neuroendocrine function could in principle point to abnormalities of neurotransmitter mechanisms in the limbic forebrain, and may be informative about the mode of action of psychopharmacological treatments. In this chapter the findings and methodological issues concerning clonidine-stimulated release of growth hormone are reviewed. Abnormal findings with this provocative neuro-endocrine probe have been described in depression and there are recent suggestions that similar abnormalities occur in panic disorder.

CLONIDINE-STIMULATED GROWTH HORMONE RELEASE

Clonidine causes a rise of plasma growth hormone (GH) concentrations in humans (Lal *et al.* 1975). Animal studies suggest that the GH response is mediated by clonidine's action on postsynaptic α_2-adrenergic receptors in the hypothalamus, to cause the release of growth hormone-releasing hormone (GHRH) into the pituitary portal system (Tuomisto and Mannisto 1985; Johnston *et al.* 1985). Clonidine also has other effects in humans. Hypotension occurs probably through postsynaptic α_2-receptors in the brain-stem; sedation may be mediated through presynaptic and postsynaptic α_2-receptors; and reduction of plasma MHPG (3-methoxy-4-hydroxyphenyl glycol) through presynaptic receptors (see Glue and Nutt 1988 for review).

Since the original report by Matussek *et al.* (1980) there have been many confirmations that the GH response to clonidine is blunted in depressed patients, especially in those classified as endogenous (Glue and Nutt 1988). Other pharmacological stimuli to GH release, such as methamphetamine (Checkley 1979) and desmethylimipramine (Laakmann 1980), are also less effective in depressed patients than in control subjects. However, the hypotensive response to clonidine is no different in endogenous depressed patients than in controls (Checkley *et al.* 1984). These findings led to the speculation that the blunted GH response to clonidine reflected 'a defect at α_2-adrenoceptors in neuroendocrine systems' in endogenous depression, though the 'defect' apparently does not involve the brain-stem postsynaptic receptors that mediate the hypotensive response to clonidine (Checkley *et al.* 1984). This speculation has never been conclusive and alternative explanations need to be considered. To do so we must first briefly review the physiology of GH control.

Control of GH secretion

The primary stimulus for GH release from the anterior pituitary gland is GHRH which, in turn, is subject to regulation by neurotransmitters in the hypothalamus. α_2-Adrenoceptor activation stimulates GHRH release, while β-adrenoceptor activation inhibits GHRH release. Dopamine can also stimulate basal GHRH release (Johnston *et al.* 1985). Furthermore, although clonidine is undoubtedly an α_2-adrenoceptor agonist, both animal and human studies suggest that it may cause GHRH release at least in part indirectly through a hypothalamic opioidergic mechanism such as β-endorphin release (Bruhn *et al.* 1989; Bramnert and Hokfelt 1984).

The main inhibitory influence on GH secretion is another hypothalamic hormone, somatostatin (SS). The release of SS is decreased by serotoninergic and cholinergic mechanisms. Conversely, SS release is increased by agents which impair 5-HT or ACh activity. The net balance between GHRH and SS determines the release of GH from the pituitary (Johnston *et al.* 1985). A short-loop feedback inhibition of GH on further release of GH has been described, possibly through increased SS release. There is also a long-loop feedback inhibition of GH release by GH-dependent peptides, the somatomedins (Johnston *et al.* 1985). These have recently been investigated in depressed patients, as discussed below.

In addition, other factors can confound the interpretation of GH-releasing challenge tests in humans. These factors include age, sex, ovarian status, body weight, weight loss, blood glucose (even within the physiological range), non-esterified fatty acids, and stress (Johnston *et al.* 1985). Time of day is another recently recognized confound. Although

Honer et al. (1984) found no difference in GH response to clonidine at different times of the day in normal subjects, more recent placebo-controlled studies indicate that time of day is important. In a study of normal short children, for example, it was found that clonidine given at 0800 h caused a definite GH response compared to a placebo injection, but that at 2300 h the GH response to clonidine was no different than to the placebo (Ghigo et al. 1990). The same is true for the GH response to pyridostigmine (Ghigo et al. 1989). Finally, it should be noted that extremely high between-subject variability is apparent in all reported studies of GH release by clonidine. This high variability complicates the task of demonstrating statistically significant differences in response between groups of subjects.

Influence of antidepressant drug withdrawal

Recent withdrawal from antidepressant drugs is a particularly important confound in clonidine–GH testing of psychiatric patients. Although Corn et al. (1984) found that desipramine discontinuation in normal subjects treated for 3 weeks reduces the GH response to clonidine for at least another 21 days, nevertheless some clinical studies have adopted shorter drug-free requirements. A recent study of this important methodological issue in depressed patients by Schittecatte et al. (1989), found blunted GH responses to clonidine in non-endogenous patients who had not received tricyclic drugs for at least 15 days (mean 16.3 days). At first glance this result would appear to contradict the report of Checkley et al. (1984) who found blunted GH responses only in endogenous depression. However, Schittecatte et al. (1989) also studied a carefully matched group of non-endogenous depressed patients who had never received tricyclic drugs. The GH responses of this group were not blunted, and were equal to those of normal control subjects. In this regard it must be recalled that the patients studied by Checkley et al. (1984) were tricyclic drug-free for at least 21 days. Thus, a minimum 3-week drug-free interval appears necessary for valid clonidine–GH testing. This requirement obviously will limit the usefulness and potential clinical application of the procedure.

Test–retest reliability

The high between-subject variability of GH responses to clonidine (and other provocative stimuli) has already been noted. A related methodological concern is the consistency of results in individual subjects. In a dose–effect study, Hoehe et al. (1988) administered 2 µg/kg clonidine IV to ten normal subjects on four separate occasions. At least one blunted GH response (peak GH < 4 ng/ml) occurred in five of the ten subjects.

Only 60 per cent of the 15 retest responses in those five patients were blunted, however. Even less consistent responses would be expected with the lower doses of clonidine (1.3 µg/kg) used in most psychiatric investigations. Indirect evidence of poor reliability comes also from another study (Brown *et al.* 1990) in which different doses of clonidine were compared. Fully one-third of nine normal subjects had lower GH responses to 1.4 µg/kg clonidine than to 0.7 µg/kg. For those three subjects the mean peak GH levels were 0.5 and 4.8 ng/ml, respectively. These results would be disturbing even had the same dose of clonidine been used in the two tests. Obviously, the standardization of the clonidine–GH stimulation test in human subjects (at least for the requirements of psychoendocrine research) is questionable.

Results in panic disorder

Against this background of methodological issues and findings in depression, we can now evaluate the studies of clonidine-stimulated GH release in patients with panic disorder. In 1986 Charney and Heninger (1986) and Uhde *et al.* (1986) reported blunted GH responses. More recently Schittecatte *et al.* (1988) found normal GH responses, with a trend, in fact, for the patients with panic disorder to have larger responses than the control subjects. The only patient found to have a blunted response had been withdrawn from a tricyclic antidepressant five weeks before the clonidine test. In the two previously noted studies (Heninger 1986; Uhde *et al.* 1986) where the GH response to clonidine was blunted, the drug-free periods were 3 weeks and 2 weeks, respectively.

In the most recent study (Nutt 1989), there was an apparent blunting of the GH response to clonidine in 13 patients with panic disorder compared with 14 control subjects. In those patients who did have a detectable GH response (6 of 13), the mean response equalled that found in the controls who had a detectable response (12 of 14). Based on these findings Nutt speculated that there may be 'subpopulations of patients with panic disorder' with regard to the clonidine–GH challenge test.

Alternative interpretations

Even if this rather weak evidence for a blunted GH response to clonidine in panic disorder is accepted, the interpretation of altered α_2-adrenoceptor sensitivity in these patients is by no means established. The blood pressure response to clonidine (mediated by brain-stem postsynaptic α_2-adrenoceptors) was exaggerated rather than blunted in two studies (Charney and Heninger 1986; Nutt 1989), leading Nutt to conclude that there cannot be 'a simple alteration in α_2-adrenoceptor function'. It is also not parsimonious to propose that the fore-brain and hind-brain α_2-adrenoceptors are differently affected, either in depression (Checkley *et al*. 1984) or in panic disorder. Other interpretations related to the known physiology of GH regulation could be proposed and have in fact been tested, at least in depressed patients.

GHRH and somatomedin

Clonidine does not stimulate GH release directly from the pituitary, but through the release of hypothalamic GHRH into the pituitary portal vessels. A blunted GH response after clonidine could, therefore, reflect pituitary insensitivity to GHRH rather than a central α_2-adrenoceptor insensitivity to clonidine. The studies of this question to date in depressed patients are not conclusive (Lesch *et al*. 1988; Laakmann *et al*. 1990; Eriksson *et al*. 1988; Krishnan *et al*. 1988). In one report, depressed patients did have a blunted GH response to GHRH 1 μg/kg as well as to clonidine, and there was a strong correlation between the two responses within subjects (Lesch *et al*. 1988). The mean drug-free period was 19 days. Laakmann *et al*. (1990) also found a blunted GH response to GHRH in male and female patients with endogenous depression, but normal responses in male patients with neurotic depression. This pattern of disturbance paralleled the GH responses to desipramine (which is also postulated to cause GH release through α_2-adrenoceptors). These two studies suggest that a pituitary defect rather than a hypothalamic α_2-adrenoceptor disturbance is responsible for the blunted GH responses to clonidine reported in depressed patients. However, Eriksson *et al*. (1988) found normal GH responses to a fixed dose of 33.3 μg GHRH in depressed patients who were drug-free for 3 months. However, they also found normal GH responses in the same depressed patients, to guanfacine (which they describe as a pure α_2-adrenoceptor agonist whereas clonidine is a mixed agonist–antagonist). Krishnan *et al*. (1988) observed normal GH responses to 1 μg/kg GHRH in 19 depressed patients, compared to a control group carefully matched for body weight as well as age and sex. There was a trend, in fact, for the depressed patients in these last two studies to have greater GH responses than control subjects to GHRH (Eriksson *et al*. 1988; Krishnan *et al*. 1988). Similarly, Thomas *et al*. (1989) found no blunting of the GH response to GHRH in 18 melancholic depressed patients compared with age- and sex-matched controls. Once again, there was a strong trend for the patients to have greater GH responses. In the one study (Lesch *et al*. 1988) that directly compared GHRH and clonidine as provocative stimuli of GH, the only apparent methodological question would concern the length of the drug-free period. From the raw data given in the report, however, it can be determined that the blunted GH responses to both stimuli were found in the subgroup of patients ($n = 6$) drug-free for over 28 days. In summary, there has never been a report on depressed patients demonstrating a blunted GH response to clonidine along with a normal GH response to GHRH in the same patients, as would be required for the 'insensitivity of α_2-adrenoceptors' theory. No studies of the GH response to GHRH have been reported in patients with panic disorder.

Lesch *et al.* (1988) also measured plasma somatomedin C concentrations and found increased levels in the depressed patients who had blunted GH responses to both GHRH and clonidine (mean somatomedin C values 1.09 U/ml, compared with 0.64 U/ml in controls, $p < 0.05$). Laakmann *et al.* (1990) also reported increased somatomedin C concentrations in endogenous depressed patients compared with controls. This finding could also be contributing to the blunted GH responses of the depressed patients to desipramine in Laakmann's study. Most recently, Rupprecht *et al.* (1989) reported that depressed patients who did not suppress plasma cortisol normally in the standard 1 mg overnight dexamethasone suppression test (DST), had much higher plasma somatomedin C (also known as insulin-like growth factor I) concentrations than did depressed patients with normal DST results.

Somatomedin C has a relatively slow kinetic response to stimulation by circulating GH (Ross *et al.* 1987). Thus, the elevated somatomedin C concentrations reported in the three studies just mentioned (Lesch *et al.* 1988; Laakmann *et al.* 1990; Rupprecht *et al.* 1989) would be expected to reflect excessive 24 h GH secretion in depressed patients. Two reports are consistent with this possibility of excessive daytime or night-time GH secretion in depression (Mendlewicz *et al.* 1985; Steiger *et al.* 1989). However, not all studies of 24 h GH secretion in depressed patients are in agreement (Rubin *et al.* 1990). No studies of somatomedin C have been reported in patients with panic disorder, nor have the 24 h GH secretory profiles been studied.

CONCLUSIONS

There is at present little reason to be confident that the GH response to clonidine in panic disorder is blunted. There is even less reason to believe that this purported abnormality would reflect an insensitivity of the central α_2-adrenoceptors in panic disorder. For that matter, the status of these two claims is not secure even in depressed patients. This review of the research literature on the clonidine–GH stimulation test illustrates several important methodological issues from which conclusions can be drawn about what needs to be done at this stage.

1. Although this provocative neuroendocrine test has been in use for over 10 years, we still have only fragmentary data on the elementary questions of dose–response relationships and test–retest reliability. Such data as do exist are not encouraging. Standardization of the test should be the first priority. Perhaps it is too inherently variable for psychoendocrine research studies.

2. The effects of psychotropic drugs and of their withdrawal need to be better characterized. Withdrawal from tricyclic antidepressants is a major potential confound of the test in clinical populations.

3. Remarkably little attention has been given to controlling other potential physiological confounds (blood glucose and non-esterified fatty acids, for example).

4. The crucial control experiments with GHRH are inconclusive in depressed patients and have never been conducted in panic disorder.

5. Somatomedin C concentrations need to be measured in all future studies to control for differences in long-loop feedback between normal subjects and patients.

Only after these questions have been settled might it be possible to claim that blunted GH responses to clonidine reflect an insensitivity of the central α_2-adrenoceptors in panic disorder, or to speculate about neurobiological similarities between panic disorder and depression on the basis of this neuroendocrine probe.

REFERENCES

Bramnert, M. and Hokfelt, B. (1984). Partial blockade by naloxone of clonidine-induced increase in plasma growth hormone in hypertensive patients. *Journal of Clinical Endocrinology and Metabolism*, **58**, 374–7.

Brown, G.W., Mazurek, M., Allen, D., Szechtman, B., and Cleghorn, J.M. (1990). Dose–response profiles of plasma growth hormone and vasopressin after clonidine challenge in man. *Psychiatry Research*, **31**, 311–20.

Bruhn, T.O., Tresco, P.A., Mueller, G.P., and Jackson, I.M.D. (1989). Beta-endorphin mediates clonidine stimulated growth hormone release. *Neuroendocrinology*, **50**, 460–3.

Charney, D.S. and Heninger, G.R. (1986). Abnormal regulation of noradrenergic function in panic disorders. *Archives of General Psychiatry*, **43**, 1042–54.

Checkley, S.A. (1979). Corticosteroid and growth hormone responses to methylamphetamine in depressive illness. *Psychological Medicine*, **9**, 107–15.

Checkley, S.A., Glass, I.B., Thompson, C., Corn, T., and Robinson, P. (1984). The GH response to clonidine in endogenous as compared with reactive depression. *Psychological Medicine*, **14**, 773–7.

Corn, T., Thompson, C., and Checkley, S.A. (1984). Effects of desipramine treatment upon central adrenoceptor function in normal subjects. *British Journal of Psychiatry*, **145**, 139–45.

Eriksson, E., Balldin, J., Lindstedt, G., and Modigh, K. (1988). Growth hormone responses to the alpha-2-adrenoceptor agonist guanfacine and to growth hormone releasing hormone in depressed patients and controls. *Psychiatry Research*, **26**, 59–67.

Ghigo, E., Imperiale, E., Mazza, E., Goffi, S. Procopio, M., Muller, E.E., and Camanni, F. (1989). Cholinergic enhancement by pyridostigmine potentiates spontaneous diurnal but not nocturnal growth hormone secretion in short children. *Neuroendocrinology*, **49**, 134–7.

Ghigo, E., Arvat, E., Nicolosi, M., Bellone, J., Valetto, M.R., Mazza, E. *et al.* (1990). Acute clonidine administration potentiates spontaneous diurnal, but not nocturnal, growth hormone secretion in normal short children. *Journal of Clinical Endocrinology and Metabolism*, **71**, 433–5.

Glue, P. and Nutt, D. (1988). Clonidine challenge testing of alpha-2-adrenoceptor function in man: the effects of mental illness and psychotropic medication. *Journal of Psychopharmacology*, **2**, 119–37.

Hoehe, M., Valido, G., and Matussek, N. (1988). Growth hormone, noradrenaline, blood pressure and cortisol responses to clonidine in healthy male volunteers: dose-response relations and reproducibility. *Psychoneuroendocrinology*, **13**, 409–18.

Honer, W.G., Glass, I.B., Thompson, C., Corn, T., and Checkley, S.A. (1984). Measurement of the GH and other responses to clonidine at different times of the day in normal subjects. *Psychoneuroendocrinology*, **9**, 279–84.

Johnston, D.G., Davies, R.R., and Prescott, R.W.G. (1985). Regulation of growth hormone secretion in man: a review. *Journal of the Royal Society of Medicine*, **78**, 319–27.

Krishnan, K.R.R., Manepalli, A.N., Ritchie, J.C., Rayasam, K., Melville, M.L., Daughtry, G. *et al.* (1988). Growth hormone releasing factor stimulation test in depression. *American Journal of Psychiatry*, **145**, 90–2.

Laakmann, G. (1980). Beinflussung der Hypophysenvorderlappen-Hormonesekretion durch Antidepressive bei gesunden Probanden, neurotisch und endogenen depressiven Patienten. *Der Nervenarzt*, **51**, 725–32.

Laakmann, G., Hinz, A., Voderholzer, U., Daffner, C., Muller, O.A., Neuhauser, H. *et al.* (1990). The influence of psychotropic drugs and releasing hormones on anterior pituitary hormone secretion in healthy subjects and in depressed patients. *Pharmacopsychiatry*, **23**, 18–26.

Lal, S., Tolis, G., Martin, J.B., Brown, G.M., and Guyda, H. (1975). Effect of clonidine on growth hormone, prolactin, luteinizing hormone, follicle-stimulating hormone, and thyroid-stimulating hormone in the serum of normal men. *Journal of Clinical Endocrinology and Metabolism*, **41**, 827–32.

Lesch, K-P., Laux, G., Erb, A., Pfuller, H., and Beckmann, H. (1988). Growth hormone (GH) responses to GH-releasing hormone in depression: correlation with GH release following clonidine. *Psychiatry Research*, **25**, 301–10.

Matussek, N., Ackenheil, M., Hippius, H., Muller, F., Schroder, H.Th., Schultes,

H., and Wasilewski, B. (1980). Effect of clonidine on growth hormone release in psychiatric patients and controls. *Psychiatry Research*, **2**, 25–36.

Mendlewicz, J., Linkowski, P., Kerkhofs, M., Desmedt, D., Golstein, J., Copinschi, G., and Van Cauter, E. (1985). Diurnal hypersecretion of growth hormone in depression. *Journal of Clinical Endocrinology and Metabolism*, **60**, 505–12.

Nutt, D.J. (1989). Altered central alpha-2-adrenoceptor sensitivity in panic disorder. *Archives of General Psychiatry*, **46**, 165–9.

Ross, R.J.M., Borges, F., Grossman, A., Smith, R., Ngahfoong, L., Rees, L.H. *et al.* (1987). Growth hormone pretreatment in man blocks the response to growth hormone-releasing hormone; evidence for a direct effect of growth hormone. *Clinical Endocrinology*, **26**, 117–23.

Rubin, R.T., Poland, R.E., and Lesser, I.M. (1990). Neuroendocrine aspects of primary endogenous depression X: serum growth hormone measures in patients and matched control subjects. *Biological Psychiatry*, **27**, 1065–82.

Rupprecht, R., Rupprecht, C., Rupprecht, M., Noder, M., Lesch, K.-P., and Mossner, J. (1989). Effects of glucocorticoids on the hypothalamic-pituitary-somatotropic system in depression. *Journal of Affective Disorders*, **17**, 9–16.

Schittecatte, M., Charles, G., Depauw, Y., Mesters, P., and Wilmotte, J. (1988). Growth hormone response to clonidine in panic disorder patients. *Psychiatry Research*, **23**, 147–51.

Schittecatte, M., Charles, G., Machowski, R., and Wilmotte, J. (1989). Tricyclic washout and growth hormone response to clonidine. *British Journal of Psychiatry*, **154**, 858–63.

Steiger, A., von Bardeleben, U., Herth, T., and Holsboer, F. (1989). Sleep EEG and nocturnal secretion of cortisol and growth hormone in male patients with endogenous depression before treatment and after recovery. *Journal of Affective Disorders*, **16**, 189–95.

Thomas, R., Beer, R., Harris, B., John, R., and Scanlon, M. (1989). GH responses to growth hormone releasing factor in depression. *Journal of Affective Disorders*, **16**, 133–7.

Tuomisto, J. and Mannisto, P. (1985). Neurotransmitter regulation of anterior pituitary hormones. *Pharmacological Reviews*, **37**, 249–332.

Uhde, T.W., Vittone, B.J., Siever, L.J., Kaye, W.H., and Post, R.M. (1986). Blunted growth hormone response to clonidine in panic disorder patients. *Biological Psychiatry*, **21**, 1077–81.

6

Panic may be a misfiring suffocation alarm

DONALD F. KLEIN

INTRODUCTION

The ability of imipramine to block both spontaneous panic attacks (Klein 1964) and panic precipitated by intravenous sodium lactate (Pitts and McClure 1967) in panic patients, suggested that panic disorder is caused by a physiological disturbance. Biological causal theories of the panic attack often posit physiological malfunctions, e.g. the locus coeruleus is excessively sensitive and erroneously discharges (Redmond 1987). Positron emission tomography (PET) has shown an abnormality in the parahippocampal region of the brain in people with panic disorder who are also sensitive to lactate infusion (Reiman 1987). Again, the idea is that the parahippocampal gyrus is part of a defective circuit that is discharging maladaptively.

The author presents a supplementary theory, which is not an alternative but considers the evolution of panic. That is, *why* should people have panic attacks in the first place? The author hypothesizes that each person has a brain integrated suffocation alarm system that decides if they are being asphyxiated, because asphyxiation is a major recurrent danger. The decision that asphyxia is likely elicits intense distress, feelings of suffocation, and the urge to flee to fresh air. Shortness of breath and dyspnea are among the most frequently reported manifestations of a clinical spontaneous panic.

Cannon's ideas about emergency emotions (Cannon 1932) i.e. the 'flight or fight' reaction, suggests that panic is a type of emergency reaction. However, novel dangers elicit discharge of the hypothalamic–pituitary–adrenal axis (HPA) (Frankenhaeuser and Jarpe 1962; Dimsdale and Moss 1980). These changes have not been observed with panic attacks in the field (Woods *et al.* 1987) or laboratory (Liebowitz *et al.* 1985a). Therefore, the spontaneous panic is distinct from the usual emergency reaction.

PANIC ATTACKS AND SODIUM LACTATE

Pitts and McClure (1967) showed that panic could be precipitated by intravenous sodium lactate in patients prone to spontaneous panic attacks but not in normal persons. Patients with other anxiety disorders are insensitive to sodium lactate (Gorman et al. 1985; Liebowitz et al. 1985b).

Patients with panic disorder often had chronic respiratory alkalosis at base-line (Liebowitz et al. 1985c). During an infusion panic, a supervening acute alkalosis was manifested by decreasing $p\mathrm{CO}_2$, as well as increasing pH.

Kelly et al. (1971) found that lactate-induced panics were blocked by monoamine oxidase inhibitor treatment in those patients who remitted. The author's group showed that tricyclic antidepressant treatment also blocked lactate-induced panic in those who entered clinical remission (Liebowitz et al. 1985c). Since chronic respiratory alkalosis disappears following prolonged panic blockade, this suggested that panic attacks are the necessary antecedent for respiratory alkalosis. However, it did not determine whether panic patients had some propensity for respiratory alkalosis, or whether respiratory alkalosis might predispose towards panic attacks.

LACTATE AND HYPERVENTILATION

Respiratory physiology tells us that, in the presence of metabolic alkalosis, which sodium lactate produces, one should breathe less, in an attempt to maintain pH by retaining carbon dioxide. What the author's group saw was that lactate infusions increased ventilation not only in panic patients but also in normals. In those who panicked, this effect was accentuated (Liebowitz et al. 1985a). Therefore, lactate exerts a pharmacological ventilatory action inconsistent with its production of metabolic alkalosis.

SUFFOCATION FALSE ALARMS AND PANIC DISORDER

The author and coworkers' initial theory was that lactate metabolized to bicarbonate, which hydrolysed into carbon dioxide and water. The bicarbonate could not cross the blood–brain barrier, but the carbon dioxide could. Therefore, the peripheral metabolic alkalosis was accompanied by a central hypercarbia and respiratory acidosis. It was hypothesized that this was the source of the ventilatory stimulation, and in panic patients, the trigger for the panic attack.

l- AND *d*-LACTATE, HYPERVENTILATION, AND PANIC ATTACKS

The biological form of lactate is *l*-lactate. The infusion given in the previously described studies was racemic (*d* and *l*) lactate. It was assumed that *d*-lactate was metabolically inactive so that it would be less likely to be a panicogen since it would not cause central hypercarbia.

The author's team gave separate infusions of racemic and *d*-lactate (Gorman *et al*. 1990). Lactate is metabolized to pyruvate, and under racemic conditions pyruvate was produced as expected. However, when only *d*-lactate was given, very little pyruvate was produced. The racemic lactate decreased the pCO_2 because of hyperventilation, but to our surprise *d*-lactate exerted a similar effect. Further, it seemed almost as effective a panicogen as *l*-lactate, although this is not definitive given the small samples. Therefore, panic was not necessarily due to the metabolic effect of the *l*-lactate but could be elicited by some non-metabolic trigger.

Lactate is unique since it comes from only one source and produces only one metabolite. Lactate comes from pyruvate during anaerobic glycolysis, which allows energy production while an oxygen debt accumulates. Therefore, increasing lactate levels suggest a relatively anaerobic situation. This occurs during exercise, but panic patients do not panic during exercise. In exercise studies (Cohen and White 1951), panic patients did not panic, but did get extremely fatigued.

The hypothesized integrative suffocation alarm centre compares multiple sources of information. Lactate increment during vigorous exercise is no cause for concern, but lactate increases without hard work, would signal hypoxia and may fire the suffocation alarm. It is suggested that this centre cannot distinguish *l*- and *d*-lactate since during evolution only *l*-lactate would have been present. Therefore, racemic lactate may be eliciting panic by two synergistic mechanisms, *d*-lactate producing a pseudo-hypoxia and *l*-lactate, both a pseudo-hypoxia and a brain hypercarbia.

CARBON DIOXIDE AND PANIC

Hyperventilation is clearly associated with panic attacks, although the nature of this association is debatable. To study hyperventilation in panic attacks, it was aimed to have panic disorder patients hyperventilate without hypocapnia and respiratory alkalosis (Gorman *et al*. 1984). This was achieved by putting them inside a balanced plethysmograph and administering 5 per cent carbon dioxide, so that they were breathing in as much carbon dioxide as they were exhaling. Therefore, hyperventilation, induced following these instructions and through carbon dioxide stimulation, did not cause respiratory alkalosis. Before the study, it was thought unlikely that they would panic under such circumstances, and it was planned to compare hyperventilation in 5 per cent CO_2 with hyperventilation in room air.

Surprisingly, the panic patients panicked more in carbon dioxide than room air. This phenomenon was previously described by Cohen and White (1951) and was forgotten. There is 0.03 per cent carbon dioxide in the air and about 5 per cent carbon dioxide in the lungs. To reiterate, the only time one would breathe carbon dioxide, during evolution, would be if forced to re-breathe ones own exhalations as would occur in a smothering situation. Carbon dioxide increment would then be the leading piece of information to elicit the suffocation response and the urge to flee.

LACTATE AND CARBON DIOXIDE AS PANIC INDUCERS

The suggestion that sodium lactate produced a brain hypercarbia, was consistent with evidence that intravenous sodium lactate caused an increase in cerebral blood flow similar to that produced by carbon dioxide (Reiman *et al.* 1989). This finding is noteworthy because very few substances beside carbon dioxide increase cerebral blood flow.

In general, however, racemic sodium lactate is a stronger panic inducer than either carbon dioxide or sodium bicarbonate. It is possible that this difference in potency is due to the fact that the components of racemic lactate, induce panic by two different mechanisms: (1) by the conversion of the lactate to carbon dioxide, and (2) by a direct, pharmacological respiratory-stimulant effect.

ACUTE HYPERVENTILATION AS AN ATMOSPHERIC TEST

Acute hyperventilation may be a test of the environment, because if a person hyperventilates in ordinary air with low carbon dioxide, partial pressure of CO_2 (pCO_2) plummets, whereas if the air is high in carbon dioxide, pCO_2 will not decrease. Hyperventilation, in a sense, is a quick analytical test to estimate whether a person is in asphyxial circumstances.

Even in patients with panic disorder who did not panic after breathing 5 per cent carbon dioxide, pCO_2 increased minute volume markedly. This finding is important because otherwise it could be argued that CO_2-exposed panic patients develop anxiety and that that is why they hyperventilate. However, these subjects did not become anxious.

RELATIONSHIP BETWEEN HYPERVENTILATION AND PANIC ATTACKS

Before panic patients received sodium lactate, but after they were already wired up and the catheters inserted, some had a spontaneous panic. This permitted the study of the panic without the confounding effect of lactate (Goetz *et al.* unpublished manuscript).

Notably, about 30 sec before panic occurred, tidal volume increased. This increase was substantially sharper and greater in spontaneous panic than in lactate-induced panic. The lactate infusion had blunted the real pathophysiological reactivity, that is the marked hyperventilation that occurs during spontaneous panic, probably by producing metabolic alkalosis. On the other hand, the increase in respiratory frequency occurs after the panic attack, consonant with a stress reaction. It is noteworthy that inhalation of carbon dioxide also causes an increase in tidal volume, and not an increase in respiratory frequency.

The panic attack appears to be a three-layer cake. The first layer is the reaction of the smothering alarm system, as if it had received an increment of carbon dioxide, by breathlessness and increased tidal volume. When the control system keeps getting signals interpreted as predictive of asphyxiation, then the panic attack, with its feelings of suffocation and urge to flee is released, followed by the increase in respiratory frequency.

This provides an explanation for the puzzling finding that hyperventilation is frequently an accompaniment of panic, but that forced hyperventilation is inadequate to produce panic. The components of hyperventilation — increases in tidal volume and increases in respiratory frequency, are complexly related to the stages of panic but are not, in themselves, causal.

CONCLUSIONS

The author suggests that spontaneous panic is a specific false alarm due to a misfiring suffocation alarm. This theory implies that chronic hyperventilation is actually protective against panic by keeping the pCO_2 well below the suffocation release threshold. The misfiring suffocation alarm theory is testable, since it implies that circumstances prone to be evaluated as potentially suffocating should increase the prevalence and frequency of panic attacks. Circumstances that make this physiologically unlikely should protect against panic.

ACKNOWLEDGEMENTS

Supported, in part, by USPHS grant MH-30906, MHCRC-New York State Psychiatric Institute; MH-33422 — Pharmacology & Physiology of Panic Disorder; MH-37592 — Psychobiology, Genetics & Treatment of Anxiety Disorders; and MH-41778 — Carbon Dioxide Challenge of Panic Disorder.

These ideas developed during the author's long collaboration with Jack Gorman, Laszlo Papp, Ray Goetz, Michael Liebowitz, Abby Fyer, Sal Mannuzza, and Rachel Klein. David Lane and Daisy Delgado performed invaluable library research and secretarial services.

REFERENCES

Cannon, W.B. (1932). *The wisdom of the body*. Norton, New York.

Cohen, M.E. and White, P.D. (1951). Life situations, emotions and neuro-circulatory asthenia. *Psychosomatic Medicine*, **13**, 335–57.

Dimsdale, J.E. and Moss, J. (1980). Plasma catecholamines in stress and exercise. *Journal of the American Medical Association,*, **243**, 340–2.

Frankenhaeuser, M. and Jarpe, G. (1962). Psychophysiological reactions to infusions of a mixture of adrenalin and noradrenalin. *Scandinavian Journal of Psychology*, **3**, 21–28.

Gorman, J.M., Askanazi, J., Liebowitz, M.R., Fyer, A.J., Stein, J., Kinney, J.M., and Klein, D.F. (1984). Response to hyperventilation in a group of patients with panic disorder. *American Journal of Psychiatry*, **141**, 857–61.

Gorman, J.M., Liebowitz, M.R., and Fyer, A.J. (1985). Lactate infusions in obsessive-compulsive disorder. *American Journal of Psychiatry*, **142**, 864–6.

Gorman, J.M., Goetz, R.R., Dillon, D., Liebowitz, M.R., Fyer, A.J., Davies, S., and Klein, D.F. (1990). Sodium *d*-lactate infusion of panic disorder patients. *Neuropsychopharmacology*, **3**, 181–9.

Kelly, D., Mitchell-Heggs, N., and Sherman, D. (1971). Anxiety and the effects of sodium lactate assessed clinically and physiologically, *British Journal of Psychiatry*, **119**, 129–41.

Klein, D.F. (1964). Delineation of two drug-responsive anxiety syndromes. *Psychopharmacologia*, **5**, 397–408.

Liebowitz, M.R., Gorman, J.M., Fyer, A.J., Levitt, M., Dillon, D., Levy, G. *et al.* (1985a). Lactate provocation of panic attacks: II. Biochemical and physiological findings. *Archives of General Psychiatry*, **42**, 709–18.

Liebowitz, M.R., Fyer, A.J., and Gorman, J.M. (1985b). Specificity of lactate infusions in social phobia versus panic disorder, *American Journal of Psychiatry*, **142**, 947–50.

Liebowitz, M.R., Fyer, A.J., Gorman, J.M., Dillon, D., Appleby, I.L., Levy, G. *et al.* (1985c). Lactate provocation of panic attacks: I. Clinical and behavioral findings. *Archives of General Psychiatry*, **41**, 764–70.

Pitts, F.N., Jr. and McClure, N.J., Jr. (1967). Lactate metabolism in anxiety neurosis. *New England Journal of Medicine*, **277**, 1329–36.

Redmond, D.E. (1987) Alterations in the function of the nucleus locus coeruleus: a possible model of four studies of anxiety. In *Animal models in psychiatry and neurology*. (eds I. Hanin and E. Usdin). Pergamon Press, New York.

Reiman, E.M. (1987). The study of panic disorder using positron emission tomography. *Psychiatric Developments*, **1**, 63–78.

Reiman, E.M., Raichle, M.E., Robins, E., Mintun, M.A., Fusselman, M.J., Fox, P.T. *et al.* (1989). Neuroanatomical correlates of lactate-induced anxiety attack. *Archives of General Psychiatry*, **46**, 493–500.

Woods, S.W., Charney, D.S., McPherson, C.A., Gradman, A.H., and Heninger, G.R. (1987). Situational panic attacks: behavioral, physiologic and biochemical characterization. *Archives of General Psychiatry*, **44**, 365–76.

7

Do benzodiazepine receptors have a causal role in panic disorder?

DAVID J. NUTT, PAUL GLUE, CHRIS LAWSON, SUE WILSON, and DAVID BALL

INTRODUCTION

The effectiveness of benzodiazepines as anxiolytics and the distribution of their receptors in brain have led to a number of theories of anxiety based on a dysfunction of these receptors. Three main hypotheses have developed. To understand these, a brief overview of current understanding of benzodiazepine receptor function is needed (for a more detailed review see Nutt 1990a). It now appears that the benzodiazepines bind to a receptor that is part of a complex of probably five proteins that act as the receptor for the endogenous inhibitory transmitter, GABA (gamma-aminobutyric acid), and also forms a membrane-spanning ion-channel that conducts anions, particularly chloride. Activation of the GABA receptor by GABA opens the chloride channel so that chloride ions flow down their electrochemical gradient. In general this flow of ions is into the cell which then becomes more electronegative and hence less likely to be depolarized. In this fashion, GABA reduces the excitability and inhibits the firing of neurones.

The benzodiazepine agonists, drugs such as all the conventionally used anxiolytics and anticonvulsants (diazepam, lorazepam, alprazolam etc.), bind to the protein complex at a site separate to the GABA receptor, called the benzodiazepine receptor (Squires and Braestrup 1977; Braestrup and Squires 1978). Binding of benzodiazepine agonists allosterically modulates the activity of GABA, so that when a GABA molecule binds to its receptor the chance of it opening the chloride channel is increased. Thus the benzodiazepines only indirectly influence chloride flux by modulating GABA action, and can be considered neuromodulators. This lack of direct action on the ion channel is in contrast to the effects of the barbiturates which also allosterically potentiate the actions of GABA, but in higher doses can directly activate the opening of the channel (Allan and Harris 1986). It is thought that this direct action can lead to the respiratory depression that is such a dangerous feature of barbiturate overdose.

Recently the concept of agonist benzodiazepines has been elaborated to encompass a class of compounds with lower intrinsic activity (efficacy). These compounds (e.g. bretazenil and abercarnil) retain anxiolytic activity, but are devoid of marked sedation in animal tests (Turski *et al.* 1990; Stephens *et al.* 1990; Haefely *et al.* 1990). Furthermore they are able to antagonize the actions of full agonists. Clinical studies with partial agonists are under way with the hope that they will be effective anxiolytics with a reduced tendency to tolerance and withdrawal.

As well as the agonist benzodiazepines already mentioned, there are two other more recently discovered classes of ligands that also bind to the benzodiazepine receptor (Fig 7.1). One class are the antagonists such as flumazenil (Ro 15-1788) and ZK 93426, which show high affinity at the receptor but have low to absent intrinsic activity (Hunkeler *et al.* 1981; Jensen *et al.* 1984; Haefely and Hunkeler 1988). These compounds block all the effects of agonists and so can be used to define the selectivity of benzodiazepines and other types of compounds for the benzodiazepine receptor (Green *et al.* 1982). The third class of compounds are called inverse agonists. These have actions which are exactly opposite to those of the agonists. They reduce the activity of GABA by decreasing the likelihood that a GABA–receptor interaction will open the chloride ionophore. Thus they reduce inhibition and this is manifest by their being anxiogenic, proconvulsant, and alerting (see Nutt 1990*a*). These actions are also blocked by antagonists such as flumazenil which demonstrates their mediation by binding to the benzodiazepine receptor (File *et al.* 1982; Nutt *et al.* 1982). A schematic outline of the receptor and the three classes of compound is given in Fig 7.1.

THE THREE THEORIES

1. An endogenous anxiogenic

This suggests that in anxiety states there is the over-production of an anxiogenic ligand (inverse agonist), that acts at the benzodiazepine receptor. Since the discovery of the receptor in brain, it has always been accepted that if an endogenous substance were acting at this receptor, it could either potentiate or attenuate the actions of the natural inhibitory transmitter GABA. The possibility of an endogenous anxiogenic was strengthened by the report that β-CCE, a β-carboline ligand for the receptor that was extracted from human urine, was anxiogenic (File *et al.* 1982). The amide analogue of this, FG 7142 was later accidentally found

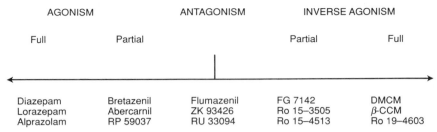

FIG. 7.1. The benzodiazepine receptor spectrum.

to cause profound anxiety in some normal volunteers (Dorow *et al.* 1983). For ethical reasons, relatively little clinical work has been carried out with inverse agonists but at least two others have been tested and found to be anxiogenic — Ro 15-3505 (Gentil *et al.* 1990) and CGS 8216 (Bieck *et al.* 1984). Interestingly there is the suggestion that this type of compound may have potential as memory/attention enhancers (Sarter and Stephens 1989), so future studies of inverse agonists in man may yet emerge. Fuelled by the early observations, several groups claim to have found endogenous inverse agonists. One suggested candidate is tribulin, an as-yet unidentified substance that displaces benzodiazepines from their receptors and whose excretion is increased in anxiety states (Clow *et al.* 1988), alcohol withdrawal (Bhattacharya *et al.* 1982), and post-traumatic stress disorder (Davidson *et al.* 1988).

Another candidate is Diazepam Binding Inhibitor (DBI). This is a peptide that displays micromolar affinity for the benzodiazepine receptor, and which has been reported to be anxiogenic (Guidotti *et al.* 1983). It may be a precursor of smaller peptides that are also claimed to display similar activities (Ferrero *et al.* 1986). If an endogenous anxiogenic was important in the causation of anxiety it could be tonically active, perhaps leading to a state such as generalized anxiety disorder (GAD). Phasic activation could lead to episodic bursts of anxiety such as those seen in panic attacks.

2. A deficiency of an endogenous anxiolytic

The second possibility is that anxiety states are caused by the relative deficiency of an endogenous anxiolytic (agonist-like) compound. There is growing evidence that such substances exist — and indeed may actually be benzodiazepines! The elegant immunohistochemical studies of de Blas and colleagues have demonstrated the presence of desmethyldiazepam and diazepam in mammalian brain (Sangameswaran and de Blas 1985; Sangameswaran *et al.* 1986), a finding soon confirmed by others (see review by Klotz 1991). Furthermore these compounds were detected in brains that had been stored from the 1940s, long before these particular benzodiazepines were first synthesized. The likely explanation for these observations is that benzodiazepines can be natural as well as pharmaceutical products. This has been confirmed by the discovery of various benzodiazepines in plants such a potato and maize (De Blas 1988). It is therefore a possibility that the evolution of the benzodiazepine receptor has occurred in response to the dietary intake of exogenous benzodiazepines in food.

It is not yet known whether those benzodiazepine agonists found in human brain can be released to affect GABA transmission. If there is an endogenous releasable agonist then anxiety might be caused by a relative deficiency of this compound(s), either tonically in GAD or transiently in a panic attack.

3. An abnormal receptor

The spectrum of activity and type of ligand at the benzodiazepine receptor, ranging from full agonist to full inverse agonist outlined in Fig. 7.1. is unique in pharmacology today. But is it fixed? Several lines of evidence suggest that it may not be, and that alterations in the 'set-point' of the receptor may be a factor in anxiety. The initial concept of a movable 'set-point' came from work on the nature of benzodiazepine tolerance. Rodents made tolerant to benzodiazepine agonists show increased responses to inverse agonists (Little *et al.* 1984). This is graphically illustrated by the production of seizures by the partial inverse agonist FG 7142 in the tolerant mice, but not in controls (Nutt and Costello 1988). In tolerance there is evidence that the antagonists become somewhat inverse in action, and by definition agonists lose efficacy (Little *et al.* 1987). Thus tolerance can be conceptualized as a state in which the receptor spectrum is shifted to the right (in the inverse agonist direction) (Nutt 1990*b*). Since anxiety is a common feature of benzodiazepine withdrawal, it is possible that such a shift in receptor 'set-point' could cause the mood state (Nutt 1990*b*).

Studies in inbred mouse strains have revealed a differential sensitivity to agonists and inverse agonists which could suggest inherited variation in the 'set-point': those sensitive to agonists perhaps being shifted relatively to the left and those sensitive to inverse agonists having receptors shifted to the right (Nutt *et al.* 1992). The genetic contribution to severe anxiety is now well recognized (Slater and Shields 1969; Crowe *et al.* 1983; Torgersen 1983), perhaps the inherited tendency is an altered receptor 'set-point' that is in the inverse agonist direction. This would tend to attenuate the actions of GABA, could lead to tonically raised anxiety, and might also predispose to paradoxical exacerbations as in panic attacks.

Hypotheses	Responses in panic patients	Responses in controls
Excess inverse agonist	↓anxiety	no change
Reduced agonist	no change	↑anxiety
Functional shift	↑anxiety	no change

FIG. 7.2. Predicted responses to flumazenil.

TESTING THE THEORIES WITH FLUMAZENIL

The availability of potent and selective benzodiazepine receptor antagonists such as flumazenil allows the testing of the three hypotheses
since each predicts clearly different responses in each case. The predicted
responses to flumazenil are given in Fig. 7.2. If an anxiogenic inverse
agonist existed then flumazenil would be expected to reduce anxiety. If an
endogenous anxiolytic were present, then flumazenil would be anxiogenic
in both controls and patients; if the receptor 'set-point' were shifted in the
inverse agonist direction, then flumazenil would be anxiogenic in patients
but not in controls.

We have tested these competing hypotheses by infusing in a double
blind randomized cross-over fashion flumazenil (Anexate — Roche) and
vehicle (Roche). This was done in ten untreated patients with active panic
disorder and ten age- and sex-matched normal controls. A dose of 2 mg
flumazenil was given IV over 1 min and the subjective and objective
responses recorded over the next hour. The dose of flumazenil was
chosen on the basis of studies by others that have used PET scanning to
estimate dose–occupancy relationships in man (Persson *et al.* 1989). These
would suggest that a 2 mg dose of flumazenil should occupy over 50 per
cent of brain benzodiazepine receptors at peak brain concentration. A
fuller description of the diagnostic and methodological aspects of the
study is given in Nutt *et al.* 1990.

The major effect of flumazenil infusion was the provocation of a panic
attack in all but two patients. Indeed every patient had a rise in anxiety
ratings, but in two these were in too few symptoms to meet DSM-III
criteria for a panic attack. The onset of anxiety was rapid, generally
peaking in the first few minutes following the infusion, and in most cases
had remitted within 30 min. Figure 7.3 shows the flumazenil — vehicle
change scores for the self-rating of anxiety, and clearly shows a significant
drug effect.

The vehicle infusion had very little action in patients and none
panicked. Both patients and volunteers were able to correctly discriminate

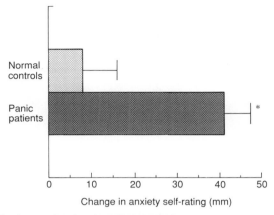

FIG. 7.3. Peak change in visual analogue scale of anxiety after vehicle infusion was subtracted from that after flumazenil infusion and the results were compared using Student's t-test. $*p = 0.003$.

the two infusions. The control subjects did not report anxiety following flumazenil, but most did describe a sense of dizziness or light-headedness that started at around the end of the infusion and lasted for a few minutes.

THE PHENOMENOLOGY OF FLUMAZENIL-INDUCED PANIC

The subjective experiences of the patients and volunteers were assessed on a number of scales, including standard 100 mm visual analogue scales and the Clark and Hemsley panic inventory (Clark and Hemsley 1982). The visual analogue ratings of individual symptoms are given in Nutt *et al.* 1990 and demonstrate significant increases in ratings of anxiety, tremor, flushing, dizziness, and racing heart. Analysis of the individual items scored on the panic inventory is given in Fig. 7.4, where they have been grouped into the different symptom classes. It is interesting that there seems to be some specificity in the responses to flumazenil, with psychological and cardio-vascular symptoms prominent, whereas respiratory symptoms showed very little change. Indeed, although most patients rated the experience of flumazenil as being similar to their naturally occurring panic attacks, several mentioned that the main difference was in the absence of respiratory symptoms following flumazenil.

Recent findings from the Psychiatry Department at the University of Leicester (see Chapter 3) have suggested that there may be two sub-syndromes of panic disorder that can be distinguished by treatment

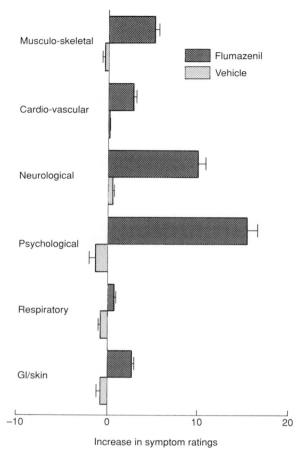

FIG. 7.4. Symptoms from the Clark and Hemsley scale were grouped together in categories. Histograms represent the total change scores from baseline (±sem) in patients with panic disorder.

response. One, defined by the occurrence of prominent respiratory symptoms seemed to respond best to imipramine whereas the other, without these, did best on the potent benzodiazepine alprazolam. This finding is highly congruent with our observation that the benzodiazepine antagonist flumazenil, preferentially provokes cardio-vascular and psychic symptoms but not respiratory ones. Together, these observations may suggest a biological differentiation of anxiety production in panic disorder.

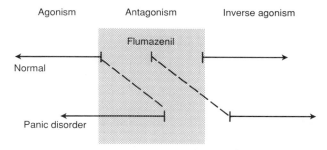

FIG. 7.5. Possible alteration in benzodiazepine receptor 'set-point'.

INTERPRETATIONS

What does the finding that flumazenil can provoke panic attacks tell us about the causation of anxiety in the light of the three prior hypotheses? It seems to us that the suggestion of an endogenous inverse agonist is no longer tenable. If one existed then flumazenil would be anxiolytic, but since it has the opposite action there can be no suggestion of even a very high affinity endogenous ligand. Thus we conclude that substances such as DBI or tribulin are not directly involved in panic anxiety.

Is there evidence for an endogenous agonist? On the face of it no — since flumazenil was not anxiogenic in normal controls. Thus there is no evidence for the view that patients might be under-producing an agonist. A subsidiary possibility does exist which still allows for an endogenous agonist, but only in panic disorder. This theory states that in order to cope with anxiety, patients turn on the production and/or release of an endogenous anxiolytic and that this compensation is antagonized by flumazenil. Hence it is anxiogenic, but only in the patient group. This theory invokes two independent processes, the production of anxiety from some as yet unidentified source, and the attempt at compensation by the production/release of an agonist. It is therefore less parsimonious than the third theory (see below) and is less explanatory of the origins of anxiety.

The third hypothesis of a shift in receptor 'set-point' is the one which gives the best explanation of the data. This is given diagrammatically in Fig. 7.5. It predicted that in anxious people, flumazenil would be anxiogenic, and indeed it was. It further predicted that flumazenil would be trivially active in normal controls and this also turned out to be the case. It is worth pointing out that there is other data supporting the 'set-point' theory of panic anxiety. The theory predicts that panic patients would be relatively resistant to the actions of benzodiazepine agonists, as they have receptors that are in a state equivalent to that seen in toler-ance. Clinical data supports this prediction. For instance it is generally recognized that to treat panic disorder with benzodiazepines, one needs to use either very potent drugs such as alprazolam, or very high doses of conventional agonists such as diazepam (Sheehan 1987; Ballenger *et al.* 1988; Noyes *et al.* 1988). Moreover there are several studies which have suggested that the performance-impairing and amnesic actions of benzo-diazepines are less in patients than controls (Malpas *et al.* 1974; Melo de Paula 1977; Oblowitz and Robins 1983). Finally, recent studies from Seattle have revealed benzodiazepine receptor subsensitivity in panic disorder. The ability of diazepam to reduce plasma noradrenaline appear-ance rate was attenuated in panic patients (Roy-Byrne *et al.* 1989), as was the reduction in saccadic eye velocity produced by increasing doses of the same drug (Roy-Byrne *et al.* 1990).

TESTING THE REMAINING THEORIES

The two residual theories are (a) altered receptor 'set-point' and (b) endogenous agonist only in panic disorder. At present there is no definitive means of distinguishing these. It is a possibility that studies with partial agonists at the benzodiazepine receptor might help. The 'set-point' theory predicts that panic patients will be relatively resistant to the actions of this class of benzodiazepines, and indeed they could behave as antagonists or even inverse agonists in these patients. In contrast if an endogenous agonist were present, partial agonists might be anxiolytic, although they could presumably also displace the natural ligand and if this were a full agonist, might also be anxiogenic. However, if partial agonists turn out to be as clinically effective as full agonists in panic disorder, then this would be clearly against the 'set-point' theory and could be taken as a refutation of it.

Another way of viewing this question is to consider the actions of full agonists. The 'set-point' hypothesis predicts that they would show reduced efficacy in panic disorder, and indeed, as already mentioned there is evidence for this. It is less clear what impact an endogenous anxiolytic agonist would have on the actions of an exogenous (therapeutically administered) agonist. One possibility is that by adding to the degree of receptor occupation, a greater activity would be produced. However, competition at the receptor with the natural ligand could apparently reduce the activity of the exogenous drug. Moreover, the presence of the endogenous agonist in patients might lead to a state of some tolerance which could itself lead to a shift in 'set-point'. Thus testing the two theories by using agonists is not likely to resolve the conundrum unless panic patients were shown to be more sensitive than controls, in which case the receptor 'set-point' theory would be refuted. This outcome is very unlikely for reasons already discussed.

FLUMAZENIL'S EFFECTS IN NORMALS

One interesting aspect of the current study is the activity of flumazenil in normal volunteers. The major effect was one of dizziness/faintness/heavy-headedness which was rated as quite marked by many, and was a major symptom in the significant increases in neurological and psychological symptoms shown in Fig. 7.4. Similar experiences were reported in 7/8 volunteers by O'Hanlon and Vermeeren (1988), who gave a 3 mg bolus of flumazenil IV. The reason for this subjective action of flumazenil is not at all clear. One possibility is that it reflects some partial agonist activity (see below) but in general, agonist benzodiazepines do not produce such a discrete and marked experience. Another possibility is that it reflects the action of flumazenil at a particular subtype of benzodiazepine receptor that the agonists do not recognize so readily. There is growing evidence for receptor subtypes based on differing subtypes of the protein subunits that make up the receptor–ionophore complex (Pritchett *et al.* 1989). Recently expression of receptors incorporating the $\alpha 6$ subunit has revealed them to have high affinity for flumazenil but not for agonists (Lüddens *et al.* 1990). Since this receptor subtype is located primarily in the cerebellum, it is quite plausible that these symptoms are initiated there.

Another intriguing observation was that of transient sweating. This was perceived sometimes by the volunteers, but was more frequently observed as a sudden deflection of the base-line of the ECG trace about 30 sec into the flumazenil infusion. The effect on the ECG is almost certainly due to a sudden increase in skin conductance caused by sweating. Similar actions of flumazenil have been reported in other studies in volunteers. For instance Higgit *et al.* (1986) found that oral flumazenil produced subjective changes that were the opposite of those found with agonists. These were increased discontent, headache, and sweating, the latter two also being observed in our study. Several other groups have also observed that flumazenil is somewhat anxiogenic in volunteers, although frank panic was not reported (Darragh *et al.* 1983; Schopf *et al.* 1984; Duka *et al.* 1986). Such responses to flumazenil are consistent with an endogenous anxiolytic ligand or with a 'set-point' in the inverse agonist direction, in those structures mediating autonomic control (headache and sweating) and mood (anxiety and discontent) in some subjects. It would be interesting to determine whether the mood changes occurred in those with a predisposition to anxiety and depression. The frequency of observed sweating appears to be independent of mood and may be the best evidence for an endogenous agonist (anxiolytic).

Interestingly Higgit *et al.* (1986) found evidence that flumazenil in some measures showed a partial agonist effect. This was seen as a reduction in EEG θ-activity, auditory evoked potentials, skin conductance fluctuations, and blood pressure. In addition the impairments of reaction time, symbol copying, and tapping rate were also in the same direction as those seen with agonists. These effects were more apparent at the highest dose (100 mg orally) which is consistent with a partial agonist explanation. In contrast Lavie (1987) found that similarly high doses of oral flumazenil were somewhat anxiogenic and delayed sleep; a much lower dose of 5 mg appeared to be agonistic in his study. Reconciling this major discrepancy is not possible at present, although the bulk of the animal evidence suggests partial agonism emerges at higher rather than lower doses (Nutt *et al.* 1982; Vellucci and Webster 1983).

There is less experience with other benzodiazepine receptor antagonists, but ZK 93426 has been given to volunteers and reported to increase alertness determined by EEG measures (Duka *et al.* 1988).

HOW IS THE 'SET-POINT' ALTERED?

If the hypothesis of an altered receptor 'set-point' is accepted then how could it come about? There is growing evidence that the $GABA_A$ benzodiazepine receptor may be changed by environmental factors such as stress (Nutt and Minchin 1983; Weizman *et al.* 1989; Biggio *et al.* 1984; Okun *et al.* 1988; Inoue *et al.* 1985; Skerritt *et al.* 1981; Havoundjian *et al.* 1986) and prior drug (benzodiazepine) experience (Little *et al.* 1987; Nutt and Costello 1988; Nutt 1990*b*). Both of these are predisposing factors in the development of panic attacks (Roy-Byrne *et al.* 1986; Pecknold *et al.* 1988; Faravelli Pallanti 1989; Lelliott *et al.* 1989). Evidence that the 'set-point' of the receptor may be different in strains of mice has already been mentioned (Nutt and Lister 1988; Nutt *et al.* 1992). There is some suggestion that inherited variation in anxiety in rats may be in part explained by differences in their benzodiazepine receptors (Robertson *et al.* 1978). Since, as already mentioned, it is well established that both genetic and environmental factors predispose to panic attacks, alterations in benzodiazepine receptor 'set-point' may be a common mechanism.

DIAGNOSTIC SPECIFICITY

An important question raised by our findings is, 'How specific to patients with panic disorder is the anxiogenic response to flumazenil?' It is important to evaluate the actions of the antagonist in other anxiety states and also in other psychiatric disorders. We have begun to do this; preliminary data in four patients with GAD suggests that flumazenil is not markedly anxiogenic in this group.

STATE OR TRAIT?

Our finding that flumazenil is anxiogenic in patients with panic disorder may suggest an underlying pathology at the benzodiazepine receptor. It does not tell us whether this might be a permanent, predisposing feature, or merely a reflection of the current state of illness, since all the subjects tested were actively ill. Studies to address this question are now under way, in that we are attempting to rechallenge subjects when their illness has remitted on treatment. So far only one subject has been willing to be rechallenged in the recovered state and she did not panic. This may be evidence that flumazenil sensitivity is state related. However since she was on imipramine at the time of testing, an alternative explanation is that this is a direct drug effect. Clearly studies on drug-free recovered patients are required.

FUTURE DIRECTIONS

To some extent these have been mentioned already: e.g. the need to examine flumazenil sensitivity in other types of anxiety disorder and in other psychiatric conditions; the potential utility of challenging with partial agonists; the resolution of the state vs trait issue. Other worthwhile projects would be the comparison of symptom and subjective experiences of flumazenil-induced panic with those produced by other means such as lactate and caffeine. Particular attention should be paid to the extent of respiratory distress.

There is also scope to explore more carefully the contribution that cognitive factors might play in the anxiety produced by flumazenil. Cognitive manipulation has been shown to modify the anxiogenic response to CO_2 inhalation (Sanderson *et al.* 1989). Indeed the safety and short half-life of flumazenil might make it a useful means of producing anxiety for therapeutic purposes; similar use has been made of lactate (Bonn *et al.* 1971) and CO_2 (Slater and Levy 1966; Wolpe 1987).

CONCLUSIONS

The finding that flumazenil is anxiogenic in patients with panic disorder has made a significant addition to our understanding of the contribution that the benzodiazepine receptors might make to panic anxiety. It now seems unlikely that this illness is caused by the activity of an endogenous anxiogenic inverse agonist. Two possible explanations for anxiety are that the benzodiazepine receptor 'set-point' is shifted in the inverse agonist direction, or that there is an endogenous anxiolytic benzodiazepine that is produced in a compensatory manner in panic patients. Resolving these competing hypotheses may be difficult, with the best approach at present probably involving the use of partial benzodiazepine agonists.

REFERENCES

Allan, A.M. and Harris, R.A. (1986). Anesthetic and convulsant barbiturates alter gamma-aminobutyric acid-stimulated chloride flux across brain membranes. *Journal of Pharmacology and Experimental Therapeutics*, **238**, 763–8.

Ballenger, J.C., Burrows, G.D., DuPont, R.L., Lesser, I.M., Noyes, R., Pecknold, J.C. *et al.* (1988). Alprazolam in panic disorder and agoraphobia: results from a multicenter trial. I: Efficacy in short-term treatment. *Archives of General Psychiatry*, **45**, 413–22.

Bhattacharya, S.K., Glover, V., Sandler, M., Clow, A., Topham, A., Bernadt, M., and Murray, R. (1982). Raised endogenous monoamine oxidase inhibitor output in post-withdrawal alcoholics: effects of *l*-dopa and ethanol. *Biological Psychiatry*, **17**, 687–94.

Bieck, P.R., Antonin, K.H., Britzelmeier, C., Cremer, C., Gleiter, C., Nilsson, E., and Schoenleber, W. (1984). Human pharmacology of CGS 8216, a benzodiazepine antagonist. *Clinical Neuropharmacology*, **7**, 674–5.

Biggio, G., Concas, A., Serra, M., Salis, M., Corda, M.G., Nurchi, V. *et al.* (1984) Stress and ß-carbolines decrease the density of low affinity GABA binding sites: an effect reversed by diazepam. *Brain Research*, **305**, 13–18.

Bonn, J.A., Harrison, J., and Linford-Rees, W. (1971). Lactate-induced anxiety: therapeutic application. *British Journal of Psychiatry*, **119**, 468–70.

Braestrup, C. and Squires, R.F. (1978). Brain specific benzodiazepine receptors. *British Journal of Psychiatry*, **133**, 249–60.

Clark, D.M. and Hemsley, D.R. (1982). The effects of hyperventilation: individual variability and its relation to personality. *Journal of Behaviour Therapy and Experimental Psychiatry*, **13**, 41–7.

Clow, A., Glover, V., Sandler, M., and Tiller, J. (1988). Increased urinary tribulin output in generalised anxiety disorder. *Psychopharmacology*, **95**, 378–80.

Crowe, R., Noyes, R., Pauls, D.L., and Slymen, D. (1983). A family study of panic disorder. *Archives of General Psychiatry*, **40**, 1065–9.

Darragh, A., Lambe, R. O'Boyle, C., Kenny, M., and Brick, I. (1983). Absence of central effects in man of the benzodiazepine antagonist Ro 15-1788. *Psychopharmacology*, **80**, 192–5.

Davidson, J., Glover, V., Clow, A., Kudler, H., Meador, K., and Sandler, M. (1988). Tribulin in post-traumatic stress disorder. *Psychological Medicine*, **4**, 833–6.

de Blas, A.L. (1988). Diazepam and *N*-desmethyldiazepam in plant food and in brain. *TINS*, **11**, 489–90.

Dorow, R., Horowski, R., Paschelke, G., Amin, M., and Braestrup, C. (1983). Severe anxiety induced by FG 7142, a β-carboline ligand for benzodiazepine receptors. *Lancet*, **2**, 98–9.

Duka, T., Ackenheil, M., Noderer, J., Doenicke, A., and Dorow, R. (1986). Changes in noradrenaline plasma levels and behavioural responses induced by benzodiazepine agonists with the benzodiazepine antagonist Ro 15-1788. *Psychopharmacology*, **90**, 351–7.

Duka, T., Goerke, D., Dorow, R., Holler, L., and Fichte, K. (1988). Human studies on the benzodiazepine receptor antagonist β-carboline ZK 93-426. *Psychopharmacology*, **95**, 463–71.

Faravelli, C. and Pallanti, S. (1989). Recent life events and panic disorder. *American Journal of Psychiatry*, **146**, 622–6.

Ferrero, P., Santi, M., Conti-Tronconi, B., Costa, E., and Guidotti, A. (1986). Study of an octadecaneuropeptide derived from DBI: biological activity and presence in rat brain. *Proceedings of the National Academy of Sciences*, **83**, 827–31.

File, S.E., Lister, R.G., and Nutt, D.J. (1982). The anxiogenic action of benzodiazepine antagonists. *Neuropharmacology*, **21**, 1022–37.

Gentil, V., Tavares, S., Gorenstein, C., Bello, C., Mathias, L., Gronich, G., and Singer, J. (1990). Acute reversal of flunitrazepam effects by Ro 15-1788 and Ro 15-3505: inverse agonism, tolerance and rebound. *Psychopharmacology*, **100**, 54–9.

Green, A.R., Nutt, D.J., and Cowen, P.C. (1982). Using Ro 15-1788 to investigate the benzodiazepine receptor in-vivo: Studies on the anticonvulsant and sedative effect of melatonin and the convulsant effect of the benzodiazepine Ro 05-3663. *Psychopharmacology*, **78**, 293–5.

Guidotti, A., Forchetti, C.M., Corda, M.G., Konkel, D., Bennett, C.D., and Costa, E. (1983). Isolation, characterization, and purification to homogeneity of an endogenous polypeptide with agonistic action on benzodiazepine receptors. *Proceedings of the National Academy of Sciences*, **80**, 3531–5.

Haefely, W. and Hunkeler, W. (1988). The story of flumazenil. *European Journal of Anaesthesiology*, **2**, 3–14.

Haefely, W., Martin, J.R., and Schoch, P. (1990). Novel anxiolytics that act as partial agonists at benzodiazepine receptors. *TIPS*, **II**, 452–6.

Havoundjian, H., Paul, S.M., and Skolnick, P. (1986). Rapid, stress-induced modification of the benzodiazepine receptor-coupled chloride ionophore. *Brain Research*, **375**, 401–6.

Higgitt, A., Lader, M., and Fonagy, P. (1986). The effects of the benzodiazepine antagonist RO 15-1788 on psychophysiological performance and subjective measures in normal subjects. *Psychopharmacology*, **89**, 395–403.

Hunkeler, W., Mohler, H., Pieri, L., Polc, P., Bonetti, E.P., Cumin, R. *et al.* (1981). Selective antagonists of benzodiazepines. *Nature*, **290**, 514–16.

Inoue, O., Akimoto, Y., Hashimoto, K., and Yamasaki, T. (1985). Alterations in biodistribution of [3H]Ro 15-1788 in mice by acute stress: possible changes in *in vivo* binding availability of brain benzodiazepine receptor. *International Journal of Nuclear Medicine and Biology* **12** , 369–74.

Jensen, L.H., Petersen, E.N., Braestrup, C., Honore, T., Kehr, W., Stephens, D.N. *et al.* (1984). Evaluation of the β-carboline ZK 93 426 as a benzodiazepine receptor antagonist. *Psychopharmacology*, **83**, 249–56.

Klotz, U. (1991). Minireview: occurrence of 'natural' benzodiazepines. *Life Sciences,* **48**, 209–15.

Lavie, P. (1987). Ro 15-1788 decreases hypnotic effects of sleep deprivation. *Life Sciences,* **41**, 227–33.

Lelliott, P., Marks, I., McNamee, G., and Tobena, A. (1989). Onset of panic disorder with agoraphobia. *Archives of General Psychiatry*, **46**, 1000–5.

Little, H.J., Nutt, D.J., and Taylor, S.C. (1984). Selective potentiation of the effects of a benzodiazepine contragonist after chronic flurazepam treatment in mice. *British Journal of Pharmacology*, **83**, 360.

Little, H.J., Nutt, D.J., and Taylor, S.C. (1987). Kindling and withdrawal changes at the benzodiazepine receptor. *Journal of Psychoparmacology*, **1**, 35–46.

Lüddens, H., Pritchett, D.B., Kohler, M., Killisch, I., Keinanen, K., Monyer *et al.* (1990). Cerebellar GABA receptor selective for a behavioural alcohol antagonist. *Nature*, **346**, 648–51.

Malpas, A., Legg, N.J., and Scott, D.F. (1974). Effects of hypnotics on anxious patients. *British Journal of Psychiatry*, **124**, 482–4.

Melo de Paula, A.J. (1977). Intravenous lorazepam and diazepam in the treatment of acute anxiety states in the neurotic: a controlled study. *Clinical Therapeutics*, **1**, 125–134.

Noyes, R., DuPont, R.L., Pecknold, J.C., Rifkin, A., Rubin, R.T., Swinson, R.P., Ballenger, J.C., and Burrows, G.D. (1988). Alprazolam in panic disorder and agoraphobia: results from a multicenter trial. II: Patient acceptance, side effects and safety. *Archives of General Psychiatry*, **45**, 423–28.

Nutt, D.J. (1990*a*). Selective ligands for benzodiazepine receptors: recent developments. In *Current aspects of the neurosciences* (ed. N.N. Osborne), pp. 259–93. Macmillan Press, London.

Nutt, D.J. (1990*b*). Basic mechanisms of benzodiazepine tolerance, dependence and withdrawal. In *Clinical aspects of panic disorder* (ed. J.C. Ballenger), pp. 281–96. Wiley-Liss, New York.

Nutt, D.J. and Costello, M. (1988). Rapid induction of lorazepam dependence and its reversal with flumazenil. *Life Sciences*, **43**, 1045–53.

Nutt, D.J., Cowen, P.C., and Little, H.J. (1982). Unusual interactions of benzodiazepine receptor antagonists. *Nature (Lond.)*, **295**, 436–8.

Nutt, D.J., Glue, P., Lawson, C.W., and Wilson, S. (1990). Flumazenil provocation of panic attacks: evidence for altered benzodiazepine receptor sensitivity in panic disorder. *Archives of General Psychiatry*, **47**, 917–25.

Nutt, D.J. and Lister, R.G. (1988). Strain differences in the response to the benzodiazepine receptor inverse agonist (FG 7142) in mice. *Psychopharmacology*, **94**, 435–6.

Nutt, D.J. and Minchin, M.C.W. (1983). Studies on [^{3}H]-diazepam and [^{3}H] ethyl-β-carboline-3-carboxylate binding to rat brain *in vivo*. II Effects of electroconvulsive shock. *Journal of Neurochemistry*, **41**, 1513–17.

Nutt, D.J., Smith, C.F., Bennett, R., and Jackson, H.C. (1992). Investigations on 'set point' theory of benzodiazepine receptor function. In *GABAergic synaptic transmission. Molecular, pharmacological and clinical aspects* (eds G. Biggio, A. Concas, and E. Costa). Raven Press, New York.

O'Hanlon, J.F. and Vermeeren, A. (1988). Effects of Ro 15-1788 on the vigilance performance of sleep-deprived men. *Human Psychopharmacology*, **3**, 267–74.

Oblowitz, H. and Robins, A.H. (1983). The effect of clobazam and lorazepam on the psychomotor performance of anxious patients. *British Journal of Clinical Pharmacology*, **16**, 95–9.

Okun, F., Weizman, R., Katz, Y., Bomzon, A., Youdim, M.B.H., and Gavish, M. (1988). Increase in central and peripheral benzodiazepine receptors following surgery. *Brain Research*, **458**, 31–6.

Pecknold, J.C., Swinson, R.P., Kuch, K., and Lewis, C.P. (1988). Alprazolam in panic disorder and agoraphobia: results from a multicenter trial. III. Discontinuation effects. *Archives of General Psychiatry*, **45**, 429–36.

Persson, A., Pauli, S., Halldin, C., Stone-Elander, S., Farde, L., Sjogren, I., and Sedvall, G. (1989). Saturation analysis of specific 11C Ro 15-1788 binding in the human neocortex using positron emission tomography. *Human Psychopharmacology*, **4**, 21–31.

Pritchett, D.B., Luddens, H., and Seeburg, P.H. (1989). Type I and type II GABA (A)-benzodiazepine receptors produced in transfected cells. *Science*, **245**, 1389–92.

Robertson, H.A., Martin, I.L., and Candy, J.M. (1978). Differences in benzodiazepine receptor binding in Maudsley reactive and Maudsley non-reactive rats. *European Journal of Pharmacology*, **50**, 455–7.

Roy-Byrne, P.P., Cowley, D.S., Greenblatt, D.J., Shader, R.I., and Hommer, D. (1990). Reduced benzodiazepine sensitivity in panic disorder. *Archives of General Psychiatry*, **47**, 534–40.

Roy-Byrne, P.P., Geraci, M., and Uhde, T.W. (1986). Life events and the onset of panic disorder. *American Journal of Psychiatry*, **143**, 1424–7.

Roy-Byrne, P.P., Lewis, N., Villacres, E., Diem, H., Greenblatt, D.J., Shader, R.I., and Veith, R.C. (1989). Preliminary evidence of benzodiazepine subsensitivity in panic disorder. *Biological Psychiatry*, **26**, 744–8.

Sanderson, W.C., Rapee, R.M., and Barlow, D.H. (1989). The influence of an illusion of control on panic attacks induced via inhalation of 5.5% carbon dioxide-enriched air. *Archives of General Psychiatry*, **46**, 157–62.

Sangameswaran, L. and De Blas, A.L. (1985). Demonstration of benzodiazepine-like molecules in the mammalian brain with a monoclonal antibody to benzodiazepines. *Proceedings of the National Academy of Sciences*, **82**, 5560–4.

Sangameswaran, L., Fales, H.M., Friedrich, P., and De Blas, A.L., (1986). Purification of a benzodiazepine from bovine brain and detection of benzodiazepine-like immunoreactivity in human brain. *Proceedings of the National Academy of Sciences*, **83**, 9236–40.

Sarter, M. and Stephens, D.N. (1989). Disinhibitory properties of β-carboline antagonists of benzodiazepine receptors: a possible therapeutic approach for senile dementia?. *Biochemical Society Transactions*, **17**, 81–3.

Schopf, J., Laurian, P.K.L., and Gaillard, J.M. (1984). Intrinsic activity of the benzodiazepine antagonist Ro 15-1788 in man: an electrophysiological investigation. *Pharmacopsychiatry*, **17**, 79–83.

Sheehan, D.V. (1987). Benzodiazepines in panic disorder and agoraphobia. *Journal of Affective Disorders*, **13**, 169–81.

Skerritt, J.H., Trisdikoon, P., and Johnston, G.A.R. (1981). Increased GABA binding in mouse brain following acute swim stress. *Brain Research*, **215**, 398–403.

Slater, E. and Shields, J. (1969). Genetical aspects of anxiety. In *Studies of anxiety* (ed. M.H. Lader), pp. 62–71. British Journal of Psychiatry Special Publication No. 3, Ashford, Kent.

Slater, S.L. and Levy, A. (1966). The effects of inhaling a 35% carbon dioxide — 65% oxygen mixture upon anxiety in neurotic patients. *Behaviour Research and Therapy*, **4**, 309–16.

Squires, R.F. and Braestrup, C. (1977). Benzodiazepine receptors in rat brain. *Nature*, **266**, 732–4.

Stephens, D.N., Schneider, H.H., Kehr, W., Andrews, J.S., Rettig, K.J., Turski, L. (1990). Abecarnil, a metabolically stable, anxioselective β-carboline acting at benzodiazepine receptors. *Journal of Pharmacology and Experimental Therapeutics*, **253**, 334–43.

Torgersen, S. (1983). Genetic factors in anxiety disorders. *Archives of General Psychiatry*, **40**, 1085–9.

Turski, L., Stephens, D.N., Jensen, L.H., Petersen, E.N., Meldrum, B.S., Patel *et al.* (1990). Anticonvulsant action of the β-carboline abecarnil: studies in rodents and baboon, *Papio papio*. *Journal of Pharmacology and Experimental Therapeutics*, **253**, 344–52.

Vellucci, S.V. and Webster, R.A. (1983). Is Ro 15-1788 a partial agonist at benzodiazepine receptors? *European Journal of Pharmacology*, **90**, 263–8.

Weizman, R., Weizman, A., Kook, K.A., Vocci, F., Deutsch, S.I., and Paul, S.M. (1989). Repeated swim stress alters brain benzodiazepine receptors measured *in vivo*. *Journal of Pharmacology and Experimental Therapeutics*, **249**, 701–7.

Wolpe, J. (1987). Carbon dioxide inhalation treatments of neurotic anxiety. *Journal of Nervous and Mental Disease*, **175**, 129–33.

8

Serotonergic basis of panic disorder

H.G.M. WESTENBERG and J.A. DEN BOER

INTRODUCTION

Disturbances in the regulation of serotonin (5-hydroxytryptamine; 5-HT) have been reported to occur in a variety of psychiatric disorders. 5-HT disturbances have been described among others in affective disorders, anxiety disorders, and aggression dysregulation.

Traditionally, the treatment of anxiety disorders has been the domain of benzodiazepines. Accordingly, the entropy of the gamma-aminobutyric acid (GABA) system, whose function is modulated by benzodiazepines, was considered to be an important factor in the pathogenesis of these disorders. But this concept, while of great importance, bears little information on the specific brain system that mediates anxiety, since GABA is ubiquitous in the brain.

Behavioural research in laboratory animals has highlighted the limbic system as the site that might be pathogenetically involved in anxiety disorders. (Gray 1982). The notion that this brain area is innervated extensively by ascending monoaminergic fibres, has called the 5-HT system into play. In the last decade a number of selective 5-HT compounds have been developed, which have increased our understanding of the 5-HT system and its possible role in psychiatric disorders.

This chapter reviews the evidence for the hypothesis that there is a link between panic anxiety and 5-HT. The relevant data supporting the role of 5-HT in pathophysiology and treatment of panic disorder will be discussed.

5-HT AND ANXIETY

Behavioural and pharmacological studies in laboratory animals have provided evidence for the involvement of 5-HT-ergic neurons in the control of anxiety (see Iversen 1984). Briefly, stimulation of the 5-HT neurotransmission, using 5-HT agonists or electrical stimulation, has been reported to result in behavioural responses (i.e. behavioural inhibition) reminiscent of anxiety. Conversely, suppression of the 5-HT system by a number of procedures would result in a decrease in anxiety. A basic problem in animal research of anxiety is that the construct validity of these models is poor. All commonly used models use the induction of 'fear' as an analogy to human anxiety, and the validation of these models is based upon their response to benzodiazepines. Hence, extrapolation from animal behaviour to various psychopathological dimensions in man is questionable.

In human, anxiety as a disorder can be divided according to the DSM-III-R-classification into four major categories: panic disorder (PD) with and without agoraphobia, social phobia (SP) and other phobias (e.g. simple phobia and agoraphobia without a history of panic attacks), generalized anxiety disorder (GAD), and obsessive compulsive disorder (OCD). The prevailing animal models of anxiety reflect by no means these different diagnostic entities. Moreover, benzodiazepines are not the treatment of choice in all four syndromes. They are commonly used in GAD, but in PD and OCD antidepressants are considered the drugs of choice.

To assess the role of 5-HT in PD, several strategies can be employed. We will focus in this review mainly on treatment and challenge studies.

THE SEROTONERGIC SYSTEM

To follow the results of the treatment and challenge studies, a brief description of the 5-HT receptor nomenclature is necessary.

The cell bodies of the 5-HT-containing neurones are located predominantly in the brain-stem. From here, ascending fibres project into distinct areas of the brain. Autoradiographic studies reveal that parts of the limbic system, especially the septo-hippocampal formation, and the cortex are densely innervated by 5-HT fibres.

In the last decade it has become clear that multiple 5-HT receptors exists in the brain. Three major subtypes of 5-HT receptors have been identified in the brain, designated as 5-HT_1, 5-HT_2, and 5-HT_3 receptors (Peroutka and Snyder 1979). More recently, they were found to be heterogeneous. The 5-HT_1 binding sites have been demonstrated to comprise at least four subtypes denoted as 5-HT_{1a}, 5-HT_{1b}, 5-HT_{1c}, and 5-HT_{1d} sites (Peroutka and Sleight 1991). This class of receptors is labelled by $^3\text{H-5-HT}$. The 5-HT_{1a} receptors are densely present in the hippocampus and raphe nuclei and are selectively labelled by 8-hydroxy-2-(di-*n*-propylamino)-tetraline (8-OH-DPAT).

Azapirones, such as ipsapirone, gepirone, and buspirone were found to mimic the effects of 5-HT on the 5-HT_{1a} sites. Electrophysiological studies have demonstrated that this receptor subtype is located presynaptically in the dorsal raphe, causing an inhibitory effect on the 5-HT neuronal firing, and postsynaptically in the hippocampus where it was found to inhibit pyramidal cell activity (Yocca 1990). 5-HT_{1b} receptors appear to be species specific; they have been identified in rat brain, but not in human brain (Hoyer *et al.* 1986*a*). The 5-HT_{1b} sites appear to mediate the release of 5-HT from nerve terminal in rat brain. *m*-Chlorophenyl piperazine (*m*CPP), the metabolite of trazodone, has been described as a potent 5-HT_{1b} agonist. The 5-HT_{1c} site was first discovered in the choroid plexus of the pig (Hoyer *et al.* 1986*b*). Mianserin was found to be a potent antagonist, whereas *m*CPP has been suggested to be an agonist at the 5-HT_{1c} site. The 5-HT_{1c} receptor appears to be closely related to the 5-HT_2 receptor in terms of structure and pharmacology; agonists and antagonists have limited selectivity between the two subtypes. Downregulation of both 5-HT_2 and 5-HT_{1c} receptors has also been shown to occur following chronic administration of antidepressants (Roth *et al.* 1989), further strengthening the similarities between the 5-HT_{1c} and the 5-HT_2 receptor. The fourth subtype, the 5-HT_{1d} receptor, is particularly abundant in the basal ganglia of the human brain. The 5-HT_2 receptors, labelled by spiperone and ritanserin, display high affinity in the cerebral cortex and the caudate (Pazos and Palacios 1985).

Very recently, Kilpatrick *et al.* (1988) identified a third 5-HT binding site, designated as 5-HT_3. Binding studies have revealed high densities in the amygdala and hippocampus of rat brains. 5-HT_3 antagonists, such as ondansetron, have been hypothesized as possessing anxiolytic activity, but the clinical data remain preliminary.

TREATMENT STUDIES

Tricyclic antidepressants

The recognition that antidepressants exert beneficial effects in panic disorder have prompted investigators to evaluate the efficacy of these drugs. The use of antidepressants in the treatment of PD originates from the observation of Klein and Fink (1962) who reported that imipramine was effective in anxiety states. The patients treated in this study were rather heterogeneous in respect to their clinical picture, but those patients that now would be classified as suffering from PD, responded favourably to imipramine. In subsequent studies they provided further evidence that imipramine could prevent panic attacks and that in most patients attenuation of panic attacks was ensued by a decrease in other psychopathological dimensions, such as phobic avoidance and anticipatory anxiety (Klein 1964, 1967).

Today several studies have confirmed the superiority of imipramine to placebo. These studies have been reviewed recently in several articles (see Modigh 1987); therefore we will not reiterate all those papers but rather address the question as to whether this anti-panic or anti-phobic effect must be considered as an epiphenomenon of the antidepressant efficacy of these drugs, or as a feature that can be explained by a specific pharmacological feature.

The point that many patients with PD have associated symptoms of depression and that these symptoms can be treated properly with antidepressants, has led to the claim that the anti-panic and anti-phobic effects of imipramine are actually an antidepressant effect. Marks *et al.* (1983) studying agoraphobic patients, all but two reporting panic attacks at some time prior to the study, found no superiority of imipramine over placebo. They concluded that the patients' low initial Hamilton depression scores might explain the absence of any drug effect, and that antidepressants may only be therapeutic for patients with dysphoric mood; however all patients in that study received concomitant behaviour therapy. On the other hand, studies on the relationship of the base-line depression score to the outcome of treatment of antidepressants in patients with PD have either revealed no correlation (Sheehan *et al.* 1980; Kahn *et al.* 1986; Mavissakalian 1987), or a negative correlation (Zitrin *et al.* 1980).

Mavissakalian and Perel (1989), by utilizing a cut-off score of 14 on the 17-item Hamilton Depression scale and excluding patients with evidence of primary or current major depression, recently confirmed these findings in that depression or depressive symptoms are not a prerequisite for imipramine's effect in PD. Moreover, recent reports that imipramine can prevent the panicogenic effects of lactate infusion in PD patients, provides persuasive evidence in favour of its specific anti-panic effect (Yeragani *et al.* 1988).

Regarding the pharmacological mechanism underlying this feature, there has been some debate as to whether the site at which anti-depressants exert the main proportion of their action is via effects on noradrenaline (NA) or on 5-HT-containing neurones.

Mavissakalian and Perel (1989) have proposed that the efficacy of imipramine in PD may be due predominantly to the 5-HT-ergic action of the drug. In a study of PD patients who received imipramine, the plasma imipramine level, but not that of the desmethyl metabolite, correlated significantly with improvement. The parent compound, imipramine, potently inhibits the neuronal uptake of both 5-HT and NA, while the metabolite, desmethylimipramine, is a selective NA uptake blocker. Thus the anti-panic effects of imipramine may be mediated through the 5-HT system.

5-HT uptake inhibitors

Studies with 5-HT selective uptake inhibitors permit one to dissect and characterize imipramine's mixed effects on these neurotransmitter systems and to explore the role of 5-HT in the pathogenesis of PD. In keeping with the presumed role of 5-HT in the mechanism of action underlying imipramine's effect in PD, beneficial effects were obtained with clomipramine and zimeldine, two selective 5-HT uptake inhibitors, in several open-label studies (Evans *et al.* 1980; Koczkas and Weissman 1981; Gloger *et al.* 1981; Grunhaus *et al.* 1984). The results of several controlled studies with selective 5-HT uptake inhibitors confirm the anti-panic and anti-phobic efficacy of antidepressants and hint at the involvement of 5-HT (Table 8.1). There is also evidence that newer drugs like fluoxetine could be effective in PD, but until now only open studies have been published (Gorman *et al.* 1987; Schneier *et al.* 1990)

To elucidate the role of 5-HT, Kahn and Westenberg (1985) studied the effects of 5-hydroxytryptophan (5-HTP) in an open study and found that panic attacks ceased in the seven patients who had experienced them. It was also noted that some patients experienced a transient exacerbation of symptoms before responding. In a subsequent double-blind and placebo-controlled study, Kahn *et al.* (1987) compared the efficacy of 5-HTP with clomipramine in 45 patients, 35 of whom met the criteria for PD. Both compounds appeared to be superior to placebo on several measures of anxiety, although the effect of clomipramine was more robust. Clomipramine and 5-HTP differed in their effect on measures of depression; clomipramine was effective whereas 5-HTP was not. A point of debate is, however, that neither clomipramine nor 5-HTP selectively affects the 5-HT system. 5-HTP, the immediate precursor of 5-HT, stimulates the synthesis of 5-HT (Van Praag and Westenberg 1983), but an effect on catecholaminergic fibres cannot be excluded (Van Praag *et al.* 1987), and clomipramine is metabolized to a desmethyl metabolite which has been shown to be a potent NA uptake blocker (Traskman *et al.* 1979).

Den Boer *et al.* (1987) compared the efficacy of clomipramine to fluvoxamine, a potent and selective 5-HT uptake blocker with virtually no effect on NA-ergic, dopaminergic, or cholinergic systems, and found both drugs to be equally effective in the treatment of PD.

Further support for the role of 5-HT in the mechanism of action of antidepressants came from a study with fluvoxamine and maprotiline, a potent and selective NA uptake blocker (Den Boer and Westenberg 1988). The mean frequency of panic attacks and the level of anxiety decreased significantly during treatment with fluvoxamine, but not with maprotiline. At the end of the trial, fluvoxamine was significantly superior to maprotiline; the latter drug had only a slight effect on the associated

TABLE 8.1. *Controlled studies with selective 5-HT uptake inhibitors in panic disorder*

Author	Diagnosis	Treatment	Therapeutic effect
Evans *et al.* (1980)	PD (25)	ZIM IMI PLAC	ZIM superior to PLA; PLA=IMI
Kahn *et al.* (1987)	PD (35) GAD (7)	5-HTP CLOM PLA	CLOM and 5-HTP superior to PLA
Den Boer *et al.* (1987)	PD (50)	CLO FLU	CLO=FLU
Den Boer and Westenberg (1988)	PD (44)	FLU MAP	FLU superior to MAP
Cassano *et al.* (1988)	PD (59)	CLO IMI	CLO=IMI CLO more rapid onset
Johnston *et al.* (1988)	PD (108)	CLO PLA	CLO superior to PLA
Den Boer and Westenberg (1989)	PD (60)	FLU RIT PLA	FLU superior to RIT and PLA

5-HTP — 5-hydroxytryptophan; IMI — imipramine; FLU — fluvoxamine; CLO — clomipramine; MPA — maprotiline; RIT — ritanserin; PLA — placebo; PD — panic disorder; GAD — generalized anxiety disorder. Number of patients in parenthesis.

depressive symptoms. These results can be taken as compelling evidence in favour of a specific antipanic effect, rather than an epiphenomenon of the antidepressant effect. The more so as depressed patients and patients with an HDRS score of 15 or more were excluded. In addition, this data provide circumstantial evidence for the hypothesis that this effect is mediated through 5-HT neuronal systems.

In several studies with 5-HT uptake inhibitors a biphasic treatment response was found: after an initial worsening of symptoms, improvement is generally seen from the third week of treatment (Fig. 8.1). This initial deterioration has previously been interpreted as a response to aversive

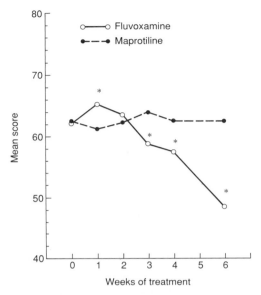

FIG. 8.1. The effect of fluvoxamine and maprotiline in patients with panic disorder as assessed with the State Anxiety Inventory. *Significantly different from maprotiline at $p < 0.01$.

stimuli, especially those elicited by the side-effects of the drugs. PD patients are thought to have augmented sensitivity to stimuli causing unpleasant bodily sensations. On the other hand, anxiogenic effects have also been observed in healthy controls during experimental stress following a single oral dose of clomipramine, but not of maprotiline (Guimaraes *et al.* 1988), suggesting that this anxiogenic effect is related to changes in 5-HT function.

Speculating about the mechanism underlying this biphasic effect, we hypothesized that the initial deterioration may be attributed to an increased 5-HT function resulting from uptake inhibition, while due to adaptive changes, e.g. downregulation, of the (post)synaptic 5-HT receptors, the clinical effects would gradually ensue. This would also explain the delayed onset of action seen in most studies with antidepressants. This hypothesis is supported by the finding that chronic treatment with most, but not all, antidepressants results in a downregulation of the postsynaptic 5-HT$_2$ receptors (Peroutka and Snyder 1980).

In summary, antidepressants which appear to exert a principal effect on 5-HT-ergic transmission, have strong anti-panic, anxiolytic, and antiphobic effects in the absence of depressive symptoms.

Ritanserin, a 5-HT antagonist

Reasoning from the hypothesis that a decrease in 5-HT function underlies the effect of antidepressants in PD and assuming that this effect is mediated through 5-HT$_2$ receptors, one would expect selective 5-HT$_2$ antagonists to be efficacious with a more rapid onset of action, because of their direct blocking effect on the postsynaptic 5-HT$_2$ receptors. To validate this hypothesis, Westenberg and Den Boer (1989) performed a placebo-controlled study with ritanserin and fluvoxamine in patients with PD. Ritanserin is a specific 5-HT$_2$/5-HT$_{1c}$ antagonist displaying anxiolytic activity in rats (Leysen 1985). Clinical studies have confirmed this effect in patients with generalized anxiety disorder (GAD; Ceulemans *et al.* 1985). The results of this study confirmed previous findings with respect to fluvoxamine, in that a significant anti-panic and anti-phobic effect was observed in the absence of formal or informal encouragement for self-directed exposure to a phobic situation. Fluvoxamine was significantly superior to placebo on several indexes of anxiety, on the frequency of panic attacks, and on measures of phobic avoidance. Ritanserin, however, had no effect on any of these measures. The results of this study permit the following conclusions. First, the anti-panic efficacy of antidepressants does not result from 5-HT$_2$/5-HT$_{1c}$ receptor downregulation. Secondly, the presumed hypersensitivity of these receptors in PD patients is not corroborated by this study. It would appear, therefore, that other 5-HT receptor subtypes, e.g. 5-HT$_{1a}$ receptors, may be implicated in the effect of antidepressants.

5-HT$_{1a}$ agonists

Recently, several agonists and partial agonists of the 5-HT$_{1a}$ receptor have become available for clinical use. These azapirones, such as buspirone, gepirone, and ipsapirone, all display anxiolytic activity in patients with GAD (Rickels *et al.* 1982; Traber and Glaser 1989; Harto *et al.* 1988). In contrast to benzodiazepines, the anxiolytic activity of these drugs has a delayed onset of action.

From two open studies with buspirone, conflicting results have emerged as to the efficacy in PD (Schweizer and Rickels 1988; Sheehan *et al.* 1988). In two controlled studies, in which buspirone was compared to placebo and imipramine, no statistically significant differences were seen among the treatment groups (Robinson *et al.* 1989; Pohl *et al.* 1989). The non-selectivity of buspirone and the huge placebo response in these studies make it difficult to draw definite conclusions. The fact that imipramine was not superior to placebo, calls the validity of these observations into question. Further studies with more selective 5-HT_{1a} agonists are warranted to further our understanding in this respect.

CHALLENGE STUDIES

To further elucidate the role of 5-HT in PD, several investigators have studied the behavioural and neuroendocrine concomitants of the acute administration of selective 5-HT agents. Particularly, the pituitary hormonal responses to direct and indirect 5-HT agonists have been used to investigate the functional state of the 5-HT system in humans. 5-HT is among the many neurotransmitters that take part in the control of the pituitary hormonal secretion. Measurement of the hormonal effects following administration of 5-HT selective drugs permits an assessment of the sensitivity of 5-HT receptor systems in the brain. There is extensive pharmacological and neuroanatomical evidence that 5-HT-containing neurones influence the hypothalamo–pituitary–adrenal (HPA) axis in rats (Fuller 1990). 5-HT-containing nerve terminals make synaptic contacts with CRH-containing cells in the hypothalamus, and direct and indirect 5-HT agonists all increase ACTH and corticosterone or cortisol release. Another pituitary hormone that is regulated, among other things, through 5-HT neurones is prolactin. There is circumstantial evidence that drugs that increase 5-HT function increase prolactin secretion as well. Using this so-called neuroendocrine strategy, Kahn *et al.* (1988*a*) studied the responsivity of 5-HT receptors in PD patients by measuring the cortisol release after administration of *m*CPP, a non-selective 5-HT agonist. When given orally (0.25 mg/kg) *m*CPP induced augmented cortisol release in PD patients as compared with normal controls and depressed patients. They also found *m*CPP (0.25 mg/kg given orally) to increase anxiety in PD patients but not in healthy controls (Kahn *et al.* 1988*b*). Based on these findings, the authors postulate that 5-HT receptors in PD patients are hypersensitive and that drugs that reduce rather than increase 5-HT function should be useful therapeutic agents in PD; the finding of Den Boer and Westenberg (1990) that ritanserin, a $5\text{-HT}_2/5\text{-HT}_{1c}$ antagonist, is ineffective in PD invalidates this hypothesis. Targum and Marshall (1989), using an oral dose of 60 mg fenfluramine, an indirect 5-HT agonist, also found significantly greater prolactin and cortisol responses in PD patients than in either depressed patients or healthy controls. PD patients also revealed a significantly greater anxiogenic response to fenfluramine administration than either depressed patients or healthy controls. These data offer circumstantial evidence that an impaired 5-HT system's dysfunctions must be considered as an important element in the pathophysiology of

PD. Other investigators, however, have debated the notion that the 5-HT/ HPA interaction is abnormal in PD patients. Charney *et al.* (1987) using 0.1 mg/kg *m*CPP intravenously, found similar cortisol and prolactin responses in PD patients and healthy controls. They also reported a similar anxiogenic effect of *m*CPP in PD patients and controls. Differences in design (dosage and routine of administration) may account for these discrepancies (Murphy *et al.* 1989). Using prolactin as hormonal probe of 5-HT activity, Charney and Heniger (1986) reported similar increases in both patients and controls after loading with tryptophan. The validity of the latter test has been questioned by Van Praag *et al.* (1987), who contend that prolactin release after high doses of tryptophan can affect catecholamine as well as 5-HT neurones. It is purported to do so by competing with tyrosine for the same carrier mechanism in the blood–brain barrier, thereby reducing the tyrosine influx into the brain, which in turn could lead to decreased catecholamine levels. Westenberg and Den Boer (1988) evaluated the responsivity of the 5-HT system in PD patients and healthy controls by measuring the neuroendocrine and behavioural concomitants of 5-HTP administration. Cortisol and β-endorphin plasma levels were used as hormonal probes of the 5-HT responsivity. Following an intravenous dose of 60 mg of 5-HTP in combination with 150 mg of carbidopa, a peripheral decarboxylase inhibitor, significant but similar increases of both hormones were found in patients and controls. Administration of 5-HTP appeared to decrease rather than to increase levels of anxiety in PD patients. Despite overwhelming gastro-intestinal side-effects, most patients had become less anxious by the end of the test. This finding also confirms the notion that exposure to adverse bodily sensations does not necessarily lead to an increased anxiety in PD patients. In contrast, controls did not consider 5-HTP administration as a relief; they developed a dysphoric mood with organic brain syndrome-like symptoms instead. Because the relatively high dose of 5-HTP and the side-effects may have obliterated differences in hormonal response, we recently conducted a 5-HTP dose–response study (Westenberg, unpublished results). Administration of 5-HTP in doses ranging from 10–40 mg elicited a dose-dependent but similar rise in cortisol and β-endorphin in patients with PD and controls. At dosages below 40 mg no side-effects were reported, supporting the idea that hormonal response was the result of 5-HTP-induced rather than stress-induced HPA activity. These findings lend no support to the presumed hypersensitivity of central 5-HT systems in PD patients.

A general problem of the neuroendocrine paradigm is the non-selectivity of the challenge agents used so far, and the complexity of the mechanisms controlling the hormones allegedly under 5-HT control.

Binding studies have revealed that *m*CPP interacts not only with all

5-HT$_1$ sites, but also with 5-HT$_2$, α- and β-adrenergic sites, as well as with dopaminergic sites (Hamik and Peroutka 1989). Many of the effects of *m*CPP in rodents, such as hyperthermia, hypophagia, hypolocomotion, anxiety-like behaviour and the elevated plasma levels of prolactin and cortisol, have been attributed to *m*CPP's agonistic effects at the postsynaptic 5-HT$_1$ receptor sites. Studies with non-selective antagonists suggest that these effects are mediated through the 5-HT$_{1c}$ receptors (Aulakh *et al.* 1987; Kennett *et al.* 1989).

There is considerable pharmacological evidence, however, that activation of either 5-HT$_{1a}$ or 5-HT$_2$/5-HT$_{1c}$ receptors leads to a stimulation of the HPA axis (Fuller 1990). In man, elevated plasma cortisol levels have also been observed after acute administration of selective 5-HT$_{1a}$ ligands such as ipsapirone and gepirone (Lesch *et al.* 1990; Rausch *et al.* 1990). In contrast to *m*CPP, these selective 5-HT$_{1a}$ ligands induce a blunted response in depressed patients (Lesch *et al.* 1990), suggesting that these effects may occur through separate pathways.

On the other hand, 5-HTP affects HPA activity through stimulation of the 5-HT release, which may interact with all 5-HT receptor subsets, both pre- and postsynaptically. It has been suggested though that the neuroendocrine effects of 5-HTP are mediated through 5-HT$_2$/5-HT$_{1c}$ receptors, since ritanserin, a 5-HT$_2$/5-HT$_{1c}$ antagonist, is able to inhibit the 5-HTP-induced cortisol secretion (Lee *et al.* 1991). The failure of 5-HTP to increase plasma 3-methoxy-4-hydroxyphenyl glycol (MHPG), suggests that central NA-ergic activity was at least not affected by 5-HTP administration (Westenberg and Den Boer 1988). These findings support the observation that 5-HT$_2$ receptors are not impaired in PD patients (Den Boer and Westenberg 1989).

In summary, the *m*CPP and fenfluramine findings are intriguing and putatively indicative of an impaired 5-HT neurotransmission in PD patients, but the present data do not permit any definite conclusions as to the role of a specific subset of 5-HT receptors in the pathogenesis of PD.

PLATELET STUDIES

Specific high-affinity binding sites for [^{3}H]-imipramine have been described and characterized on human platelet membranes (Paul *et al.* 1980). These binding sites appear similar to the [^{3}H]-imipramine binding sites found in the human brain, and there is circumstantial evidence that these sites are associated with, but not identical to, the 5-HT uptake mechanism in both platelets and neurones (Langer *et al.* 1980). It has been suggested therefore that [^{3}H]-imipramine binding labels a physiologically relevant site that modulates 5-HT reuptake. A reduction in the maximum concentration or density of platelet [^{3}H]-imipramine binding sites has been reported in depressed patients by some investigators (Paul *et al.* 1981; Raisman *et al.* 1981; Roy *et al.* 1987; Innis *et al.* 1987).

Studies conducted so far in patients with PD do not reveal abnormal [^{3}H]-imipramine binding characteristics (Norman *et al.* 1986; Innis *et al.* 1987; Nutt and Fraser 1987; Schneider *et al.* 1987; Uhde *et al.* 1987; Norman and Sartor 1989). In spite of the fact that the number of subjects was relatively small in all studies, it can be concluded that [^{3}H]-imipramine binding in PD patients is normal, thus possibly pointing to a different pathogenesis of depression and PD.

In a recent study, a decreased number of [^{3}H]-LSD binding sites on the platelet membrane of PD patients as compared to controls was found (Norman *et al.* 1990).

Platelet 5-HT uptake is also considered to share several properties with the presynaptic terminal of 5-HT-containing fibres, and is therefore used as a peripheral probe of the presynaptic 5-HT function in the brain (Stahl *et al.* 1982).

Platelet 5-HT uptake has been reported to be lowered among depressed patients (Tuomisto and Tukiainen 1976; Meltzer *et al.* 1984). In two studies an augmented maximal uptake rate (V_{max}) and a similar K_m was found in patients with PD relative to healthy controls (Norman *et al.* 1986, Noum & Sartor 1989). In contrast, Pecknold *et al.* (1988) found a reduced V_{max} in patients with PD, whereas Den Boer and Westenberg (1990) found no difference in the platelet kinetics between patients with PD and healthy controls.

Taking these data together, one might conclude that these peripheral indices of 5-HT function do not disclose any 5-HT abnormality in PD. They might point, however, to a pathogenic difference between PD and depression. The finding of a reduced [^{3}H]-LSD binding is also in contrast to the postulated supersentitivity of the postsynaptic 5-HT$_2$ receptors in PD.

DISCUSSION

The most pertinent finding to emerge from these studies is the effect of 5-HT uptake inhibitors in PD patients. The biphasic profile of these drugs in PD patients and the late onset of action (Fig. 8.1) were taken as evidence for alterations in the 5-HT receptor function. In line with the animal data, it has been hypothesized that the initial exacerbation of symptoms is accounted for by stimulation of the 5-HT system, resulting from uptake inhibition. The subsequent anti-panic and anxiolytic effects could be explained by the compensatory downregulation of the 5-HT receptors. The augmented neuroendocrine responses and pro-anxiogenic effects of mCPP and fenfluramine seen by some investigators seem to support this theory. Yet there are a number of contradictory findings so that these findings should be interpreted with certain caution. Moreover, these challenge studies were performed with pharmacological agents that are extremely non-selective. Therefore, it is difficult to attribute the effects of mCPP and fenfluramine to an interaction with a specific 5-HT receptor subtype.

Furthermore, the hypothesis that a subtype of 5-HT receptors might be supersensitive in PD rests upon the presumption that acute treatment with 5-HT uptake inhibitor results in an enhanced 5-HT function, while long-term treatment leads to a reduced 5-HT neurotransmission.

At variance with this assumption, electrophysiological studies have revealed that long-term treatment with 5-HT uptake blockers lead to an enhanced 5-HT neurotransmission through 5-HT autoreceptor down-regulation (De Montigny and Aghajanian, 1978; Chaput *et al.* 1988). These studies reveal that acute treatment with 5-HT uptake blockers reduces the 5-HT neuronal impulse flow. This somewhat unexpected finding has been attributed to an increased activation of the 5-HT$_{1a}$ autoreceptors that reside on the cell bodies of the 5-HT-containing neurones, resulting in a reduced 5-HT neurotransmission in the hippocampus. Long-term administration with 5-HT uptake inhibitors significantly reduced the 5-HT$_{1a}$ binding sites in the dorsal raphe (Welner *et al.* 1989). Moret and Briley (1990), studying the *in-vitro* release of 5-HT, found that treatment with citalopram, a selective 5-HT uptake inhibitor, for 21 days resulted in a downregulation of the 5-HT terminal autoreceptor in rat brain slices. In congruence with these findings, electrophysiological reports indicate a desensitization of the somatodendritic and terminal 5-HT autoreceptors following long-term treatment with 5-HT uptake blockers (Chaput *et al.* 1986; Blier *et al.* 1988). Desensitization of these autoreceptors would permit these neurones to restore their normal firing rate, resulting in a net gain in efficacy of synaptic transmission. If this reasoning is correct, one would predict symptoms of anxiety and panic to be associated with a decreased rather than an increased 5-HT function in brain areas controlling anxiety, e.g. the septo-hippocampal formation.

Interestingly, acute and long-term treatment with gepirone, a selective 5-HT$_{1a}$ agonist, mimicked the effects of the 5-HT uptake blockers (Blier and De Montigny 1990). Thus, the 5-HT$_{1a}$ agonists appear to possess the 5-HT modifying characteristics of antidepressants. Hence, these drugs deserve further clinical testing in PD patients both after acute and chronic administration. Such studies may help to elucidate the specific neurochemical events underlying the treatment and pathophysiology of PD. In view of the complexity of the anatomical and functional interactions between 5-HT and other neuronal systems in the brain, most notably the NA system, it seems apparent that no single theory can account for all the events provoked by antidepressants in man. Moreover, processes beyond the 5-HT receptor must be taken into account as well.

REFERENCES

Aulakh, C.S., Cohen, R.M., Hill, J.L., Murphy, D.L., and Zohar, J. (1987). Long-term imipramine treatment enhances locomotor and food intake suppressant effects of *m*-chlorophenylpiperazine in rats. *British Journal of Pharmacology*, **91**, 747–52.

Blier, P., De Montigny, C., and Chaput, Y. (1988). Electrophysiological assessment of the effects of antidepressant treatments on the efficacy of 5-HT neurotransmission. *Clinical Neuropharmacology*, **11**, 1S–10S.

Blier, P. and De Montigny, C. (1990). Differential effect of gepirone on presynaptic and postsynaptic serotonin receptors: single-cell recording studies. *Journal of Clinical Psychopharmacology*, **10**, 13S–20S.

Cassano, G.B., Petracca, A., Perugi, G., Nisista, C., Musetti, L., Mengali, F., McNair, D.M. (1988). Clomipramine for panic disorder: I. The first 10 weeks of a long-term comparison with imipramine. *Journal of Affective Disorders*, **14**, 123–7.

Ceulemans, D.L.S., Hoppenbrouwers, M.L.J.A., Gelders, Y.G., and Reyntjens, A.J.M. (1985). The influence of ritanserin, a serotonergic antagonist, in anxiety disorders: a double-blind placebo-controlled study versus lorazepam. *Pharmacopsychiatry*, **8**, 303–5.

Chaput, Y., De Montigny, C., and Blier, P. (1986). Effects of selective 5-HT uptake blocker, citalopam, on the sensitivity of the 5-HT autoreceptor. Electrophysiological studies in the rat brain. *Naunyn-Schmiedeberg's Archive of Pharmacology*, **333**, 342–8.

Chaput, Y., Blier, P., and De Montigny, C. (1988). Acute and long-term effects of antidepressant serotonin (5-HT) uptake blockers on the efficacy of 5-HT neurotransmission. Electrophysiological studies in the rat central nervous system. *Advances in Biological Psychiatry*, **17**, 1–17.

Charney, D.S., Woods, S.W., Goodman, W.K., and Heninger, G.R. (1987). Serotonin function in anxiety. *Psychopharmacology*, **92**, 14–24.

Charney, D.S. and Heninger, G.R. (1986). Serotonin function in panic disorders. *Archives of General Psychiatry*, **43**, 1059–65.

de Montigny, C. and Aghajanian, G.K. (1978). Tricyclic antidepressants: long-term treatment increases responsivity of rat forebrain neurons to serotonin. *Science*, **202**, 1303–6.

Den Boer, J.A., Westenberg, H.G.M., Kamerbeek, W.D.J., Verhoeven, W.M.A., and Kahn, R.S. (1987). Effect of serotonin uptake inhibitors in anxiety disorders, a double-blind comparison of clomipramine and fluvoxamine. *International Journal of Clinical Psychopharmacology*, **2**, 21–32.

Den Boer, J.A. and Westenberg, H.G.M. (1988). Effect of a serotonin and noradrenaline uptake inhibitor in panic disorder, a double-blind comparative study with fluvoxamine and maprotiline. *International Journal of Clinical Psychopharmacology*, **3**, 59–74.

Den Boer, J.A. and Westenberg, H.G.M. (1990). Serotonin function in panic disorder: a double blind placebo controlled study with fluvoxamine and ritanserin. *Psychopharmacology*, **102**, 85–94.

Evans, L., Best, J., Moore, G., and Cox, J. (1980). Zimeldine- a serotonin uptake blocker in the treatment of phobic anxiety. *Progress in Neuro-Psychopharmacology and Biological Psychiatry*, **4**, 75–9.

Fuller, W. (1990). Serotonin receptors and neuroendocrine responses. *Neuropsychopharmacology*, **3**, 495–502.

Gloger, S., Grunhaus, L., Birmacher, B., and Troudart, T. (1981). Treatment of spontaneous panic attacks with clomipramine. *American Journal of Psychiatry*, **138**, 1215–17.

Gorman, J.M., Liebowitz, M.R., Feyer, A.J., Goetz, D., Campaes, R.B. Feyer, M.J. *et al.* (1987). An open trial of fluoxetine in the treatment of panic attacks, *Journal of Clinical Psychopharmacology*, **7**, 329–32.

Gray, J.A. (1982). *The neuropsychology of anxiety*. Oxford University Press, Oxford.

Grunhaus, L., Gloger, S., and Birmacher, B. (1984). Clomipramine treatment for panic attacks in patients with mitral valve prolapse. *Journal of Clinical Psychiatry*, **45**, 25–7.

Guimaraes, F.S., Zuardi, A.W., and Graeff, F.G. (1988). Effect of chlorimipramine and maprotiline on experimental anxiety in humans. *Journal of Psychopharmacology*, **1**, 184–92.

Hamik, A. and Peroutka, S.J. (1989). 1-(m-Chlorophenyl) piperazine (mCPP) Interactions with neurotransmitter receptors in the human brain. *Biological Psychiatry*, **25**, 569–75.

Harto, N.E., Branconnier, R.J., Spera, K.F., and Dessain, E.C. (1988). Clinical profile of gepirone, a nonbenzodiazepine anxiolytic. *Psychopharmacology Bulletin*, **24**, 154–60.

Hoyer, D., Pazos, A., Probst, A., and Palacios, J.M. (1986a). Serotonin receptors in the human brain. I Characterization and autoradiographic localization of 5-HT$_{1a}$ recognition sites. Apparent absence of 5-HT$_{1b}$ recognition sites. *Human Brain Research*, **376**, 85–96.

Hoyer, D., Pazos, A., Probst, A., and Palacios, J.M. (1986b). Serotonine receptors in the human brain. II Characterization and autoradiographic localization of 5-HT$_{1c}$ and 5-HT$_2$ recognition Sites. *Brain Research*, **376**, 97–107.

Innis, R.B., Charney, D.S., and Heninger, G.R., (1987). Differential ^{3}H-imipramine platelet binding in patients with panic disorder and depression. *Psychiatry Research*, **21**, 33–41.

Iversen, D.S. (1984). 5-HT and anxiety. *Neuropharmacology*, **23**, 1553–60.

Johnston, D.G., Troyer, I.E., and Whitstett, S.F. (1988). Clomipramine in the treatment of agoraphobic women. *Biological Psychiatry*, **25**, 101–4.

Kahn, R.S. and Westenberg, H.G.M. (1985). L-5-Hydroxytryptophan in the treatment of anxiety disorders. *Journal of Affective Disorders*, **8**, 197–200.

Kahn, R.S., Asnis, G.M., Wetzler. S., and Van Praag, H.M. (1988a). Neuroendocrine evidence for serotonin receptor hypersensitivity in panic disorder. *Psychopharmacology*, **96**, 360–4.

Kahn, R.S., Welzer, S., Van Praag, H.M., Asnis, G.M., and Strauman, T. (1988*b*). Behavioral indications for serotonin receptor hypersensitivity in panic disorder. *Psychiatry Research*, **25**, 101–4.

Kahn, R.S., Westenberg, H.G.M., Verhoeven, W.M.A., Gispen-de Wied, C.C., and Kamerbeek, W.D.J. (1987). Effect of a serotonin precursor and uptake inhibitor in anxiety disorders, a double-dlind comparison of 5-hydroxytryptophan, clomipramine and placebo. *International Journal of Clinical Psychopharmacology*, **2**, 33–45.

Kahn, R.J., McNair, D.M. Lipman, R.S., Covi, L., Rickels, K., Downing, R. *et al.* (1986). Imipramine and chlordiazepoxide in depressive and anxiety disorders. *Archives of General Psychiatry*, **43**, 79–85.

Kennett, G.A., Whitton, P., Shah, K., and Curzon, G. (1989). Anxiogenic-like effects of *m*CPP and TFMPP in animal models are opposed by 5-HT$_{1C}$ receptor antagonists. *European Journal of Pharmacology*, **164**, 445–54.

Kilpatrick, G.J., Jones, B.J., and Tyers, M.B. (1988). Identification and distribution of 5-HT$_3$ receptors in rat brain using radioligand binding. *Nature*, **330**, 746–8.

Klein, D.F. (1964). Delineation of two drug-responsive anxiety syndromes. *Psychopharmacologia*, **5**, 397–408.

Klein, D.F. (1967). The importance of psychiatric diagnosis in pediction of clinical drug effects. *Archives of General Psychiatry*, **16**, 118–26.

Klein, D.F. and Fink, M. (1962). Psychiatric reaction patterns to imipramine. *American Journal of Psychiatry*, **119**, 432–8.

Koczkas, S. and Weissman, A. (1981). A pilot study of the effect of the 5-HT-uptake inhibitor, zimeldine, on phobic anxiety. *Acta Psychiatrica Scandinavica*, **290**, 328–341.

Langer, S.Z., Moret, C., Raisman, R., Dubocovitch, M., and Briley, M. (1980). High affinity ^{3}H-imipramine binding in rat hypthalamus: association with uptake of serotonin but not norepinephrine. *Science*, **210**, 1133–5.

Lee, M.A., Nash, J.F., Barnes, M., and Meltzer, H.Y. (1991). Inhibitory effect of ritanserin on the 5-hydroxytryptophan-mediated cortisol, ACTH and prolactine secretion in humans. *Psychopharmacology*, **103**, 258–64.

Lesch, K.P., Mayer, S., Disslekamp-Tietze, J., Hoh, A., Wieman, M., Osterheider *et al.* (1990). 5-HT$_{1a}$ receptor responsivity in unipolar depression. Evaluation of ipsapirone-induced ACTH and cortisol secretion in patients and controls. *Biological Psychiatry*, **28**, 620–8.

Leysen, J.E. (1985). Characterization of serotonin receptor binding sites. In *Neuropharmacology of serotonin* (ed. A.E. Geen), pp. 79–114. Oxford University Press.

Marks, I.M., Gray, S., Cohen, D., Hill, R., Mawson, D., Ramm, E. *et al.* (1983). Imipramine and brief therapist-aided exposure in agoraphobics having self-exposure homework. *Archives of General Psychiatry*, **40**, 153–62.

Mavissakalian, M. (1987). Initial depression and response to imipramine in agoraphobia. *Journal of Nervous and Mental Disease*, **175**, 358–61.

Mavissakalian, M. and Perel, J.M. (1989). Imipramine dose–response relationship in panic disorder with agoraphobia. *Archives of General Psychiatry*, **46**, 127–31.

Meltzer, H.Y., Lowy, M., Robertson, A., Goodnick, P., and Perline, R. (1984). Effect of 5-hydroxytryptophan on serum cortisol level in major affective disorders. *Archives of General Psychiatry*, **41**, 391–7.

Modigh, K. (1987). Antidepressant drugs in anxiety disorders. *Acta Psychiatrica Scandinavica*, **76** (suppl. 335), 57–71.

Moret, C. and Briley, M. (1990). Serotonin autoreceptor subsensitivity and antidepressant activity. *European Journal of Pharmacology*, **180**, 351–6.

Murphy, D.L., Mueller, E.A., Hill, J.L., Tolliver, T.J., and Jacobsen, F.M. (1989). Comparative anxiogenic, neuroendocrine, and physiological effects of *m*-clorophenylpiperazine given intravenously or orally to healthy volunteers. *Psychopharmacology*, **98**, 275–83.

Norman, T.R. and Sartor, D.M. (1989). Platelet serotonin uptake and ^{3}H-imipramine binding in panic disorder. *Journal of Affective Disorders*, **17**, 77–81.

Norman, T.R., Judd, F.K., Gregory, M. *et al.* (1986). Platelet serotonin uptake in panic disorder. *Journal of Affective Disorders*, **11**, 69–72.

Norman, T.R., Judd, F.K., Staikos, V., Burrows, C.D., and McIntyre, I.M. (1990). High-affinity platelet [3H] LSD binding is decreased in panic disorder. *Journal of Affective Disorders*, **19**, 119–23.

Nutt, D.J. and Fraser, Sh. (1987). Platelet binding studies in panic disorder. *Journal of Affective Disorders*, **12**, 7–11.

Paul, S.M., Rehavi, M., Skolnick, K.P., Ballenger, J.C., and Goodwin, K. (1981). Depressed patients have decreased binding of tritiated imipramine to platelet serotonin transporter. *Archives of General Psychiatry*, **38**, 1315–17.

Paul, S.M., Rehavi, M., Skolnick, P., and Goodwin, F.K. (1980). Demonstration of high-affinity binding sites for ^{3}H-imipramine on human platelets. *Life Sciences*, **26**, 953–9.

Pazos, A. and Palacios, J.M. (1985). Quantitative autoradiographic mapping of serotonin receptors in rat brain. I. Serotonin-I receptors. *Brain Research*, **346**, 205–30.

Pecknold, J.C., Suranyi-Cadotte, B., Chang, H. and Nair, N.P.V. (1988). Serotonin uptake in panic disorder and agoraphobia. *Neuropsychopharmacology*, **39**, 917–28.

Peroutka, S.J. and Snyder, S.H. (1979). Multiple serotonin receptors: differential binding of ^{3}H-serotonin, ^{3}H-lysergic acid diethylamide and ^{3}H-spiroperidol. *Molecular Pharmacology*, **16**, 687–99.

Peroutka, S.J. and Snyder, S.H. (1980). Long term antidepressant treatment decreases spiroperidol labeled serotonin receptor binding. *Science* **210**, 88–90.

Peroutka, S.J. and Sleight, A.J. (1991). Central serotonin receptors. Functional correlates and clinical relevance. In *The role of serotonin in psychiatric disorders* (ed. S.L. Brown and H.M. Van Praag), pp. 8–26. Brunnel and Mazel, New York.

Pohl, R., Balon, R., Yeragani, V.K., and Gershon, S. (1989). Serotonergic anxiolytics in the treatment of panic disorder: a controlled study with buspirone. *Psychopathology*, **22** (suppl. 1), 60–7.

Raisman, R., Sechter, D., Briley, M.S., Zarifian, E., and Langer, S.Z. (1981). High affinity ^{3}H-imipramine binding in platelets from untreated and treated depressed patients compared to healthy volunteers. *Psychopharmacology*, **75**, 368–71.

Rausch, J.L., Stahl, S.M., and Hauger, R. (1990). Cortisol and growth hormone responses to the 5-HT$_{1a}$ agonist gepirone in depressed patients. *Biological Psychiatry*, **28**, 73–8.

Rickels, K., Weisman, K., Norstad, N., Singer, M., Stoltz, D., Brown, A. *et al.* (1982). Buspirone and diazepam in anxiety: a controlled study. *Journal of Clinical Psychiatry*, **43**, 81–86.

Robinson, D.R., Shrotriya, R.C., Alms, D.R., Messina, M., and Andary, J. (1989). Treatment of panic disorder: nonbenzodiazepine anxiolytics, including buspirone. *Psychopharmacology Bulletin*, **25**, 21–6.

Roth, B.L., Decker, L., and Herkenham, M. (1989). An autoradiographic study of mianserin-induced down regulation of serotonin (5-HT$_2$ and 5-HT$_{1c}$) receptors. *Biological Psychiatry*, **25**, 42A.

Roy, A., Everett, D., Pickar, D., and Paul, S.M. (1987). Platelet tritiated imipramine binding and serotonin uptake in depressed patients and controls: relationship between plasma cortisol levels before and after dexemethason administration. *Archives of General Psychiatry*, **44**, 320–7.

Schneider, L.S., Munjack, D., Severson, J.A., and Palmer, R. (1987). Platelet [³H] imipramine binding in generalized anxiety disorder, panic disorder and agoraphobia with panic attacks. *Biological Psychiatry*, **22**, 59–66.

Schneier, F.R., Liebowitz, M.R., Davies, S.O., Fairbanks, J., Hollander, E., Campeas, R. *et al.* (1990). Fluoxetine in panic disorder. *Journal of Clinical Psychopharmacology*, **10**, 119–21.

Schweizer, E. and Rickels, K. (1988). Buspirone in the treatment of panic disorder: a controlled pilot comparison with clorazepate. *Journal of Clinical Psychopharmacology*, **8**, 303.

Sheehan, D.V., Ballenger, J., and Jacobsen, G. (1980). Treatment of endogenous anxiety with phobic, hysterical and hypochodriacal symptoms. *Archives of General Psychiatry*, **37**, 51–9.

Sheehan, D.V., Raj, A.B., Sheehan, K.H., and Soto, S. (1988). The relative efficacy of buspirone, imipramine and placebo in panic disorder: a preliminary report. *Pharmacology, Biochemistry and Behavior*, **29**, 815–17.

Stahl, S.M., Ciaranello, R.D., and Berger, P.A. (1982). Platelet serotonin in schizophrenia and depression. In *Serotonin in Biological Psychiatry* (ed. B.T. Ho) pp. 182. Raven Press, New York.

Targum, S.D. and Marshall, L.E. (1989). Fenfluramine provocation of anxiety in patients with panic disorder, *Psychiatry Research*, **28**, 295–306.

Traber, J. and Glaser, Th. (1987). 5-HT1a receptor-related anxiolytics. *TIPS*, **8**, 432–7.

Traskman, L., Asberg, M., and Bertilsson, L. (1979). Plasma levels of chlorimipramine and its desmethyl metabolite during treatment of depression. *Clinical Pharmacology and Therapeutics*, **26**, 600–69.

Tuomisto, J. and Tukiainen, E. (1976). Depressed uptake of 5-hydroxytryptamine in blood platelets from depressed patients. *Nature*, **262**, 596–8.

Uhde, T.W., Berrettini, W.H., Boy-Byrne, P.P., Boulenger, J. Ph., and Post, R.M.

(1987). [³H]Imipramine binding in patients with panic disorder. *Biological Psychiatry*, **22**, 52–8.

Van Praag, H.M. and Westenberg, H.G.M. (1983). The treatment of depression with 1-5-hydroxytryptophan. In *Treatment of depression with monoamine precursors*, (ed. H.M. van Praag and J. Mendlewicz), pp. 94–128. Karger, Basel.

Van Praag, H.M., Lemus, C., and Kahn, R.S. (1987). Hormonal probes of central serotonergic activity: do they really exist? *Biological Psychiatry*, **22**, 86–98.

Welner, S.A., De Montigny, C., Desroches, J., Desjardin, P., and Suranyi-Cadotte, B.E. (1989). Autoradiographic quantification of serotonin (5-HT$_{1a}$) receptors following long-term antidepressant treatment. *Synapse*, **4**, 347–53.

Westenberg, H.G.M. and Den Boer, J.A. (1989). Selective monoamine uptake inhibitors and a serotonin antagonist in the treatment of panic disorder. *Psychopharmacology Bulletin*, **25**, 119–23.

Yeragani, V.K., Pohl, R., Balon, R., Rainey, J.M., Berchou, R., and Ortiz, A. (1988). Sodium lactate infusion after treatment with tricyclic antidepressants: behavioral and physiological findings. *Biological Psychiatry*, **24**, 767–74.

Yocca, F.D. (1990). Neurochemistry and neurophysiology of buspirone and gepirone: interactions at the pressynaptic and postsynaptic 5-HT$_{1a}$ receptors. *Journal of Clinical Psychopharmacology*, **10**, 6S–12S.

Zitrin, C.M., Klein, D.F., and Woerner, M. (1980). Treatment of agoraphobia with group exposure *in vivo* and imipramine. *Archives of General Psychiatry*, **37**, 63–72.

9

Cholecystokinin and panic disorders

JACQUES BRADWEJN, DIANA KOSZYCKI, RICHARD PAYEUR, and MICHEL BOURIN

INTRODUCTION

The neurobiology of panic disorders is unknown. Evidence suggests that panic attacks may be triggered by a central nervous system dysfunction in mid-brain structures that involve noradrenergic and serotoninergic neurotransmitter systems. Exhaustive reviews of these theories appear in several publications (Gorman *et al.* 1989; Redmond 1987).

The use of provocative agents (i.e. lactate, CO_2, yohimbine, isoproterenol) represents a viable way of investigating the biochemical and physiological events that occur during a panic attack (Gorman *et al.* 1987). It is hoped that these agents will help uncover the neurobiological systems associated with the etiology of panic attacks. It is likely that several neurochemical systems act concurrently and sequentially to produce an attack.

The development of provocative agents which affect neurochemical systems selectively and at a specific locus in a chain of neurochemical events, might help elucidate the neurobiological basis of panic attacks and related disorders. For instance, the panicogen yohimbine has been associated with α_2-adrenoceptors by decreasing negative feedback inhibition which activates impulse flow and noradrenergic (NA) release (Grant and Redmond 1981; Maas *et al.* 1977), whereas other agents (for example sodium lactate, CO_2) have not demonstrated a clear association with any system. The increased use in research of a variety of panic-inducing agents has prompted researchers to establish specific criteria for an ideal provocative agent (Guttmacher *et al.* 1983; Gorman *et al.* 1987). Recent empirical data in humans indicate that the tetrapeptide form of cholecystokinin (CCK-4) satisfies criteria for a panicogenic agent for research in panic disorder (Bradwejn *et al.* 1991).

CHOLECYSTOKININ AND THE CENTRAL NERVOUS SYSTEM

Cholecystokinin (CCK) is a peptide found in high density in the cerebral cortex, the amygdala and the hippocampus of the mammalian brain (Roberts *et al.* 1982; Beinfeld 1983; Reeve *et al.* 1984). Molecular forms of varying amino acid lengths of CCK have been isolated. The sulphated octapeptide (CCK-8S) is the most abundant form, and shorter molecular forms are also present in the brain (Sauter and Frick 1983; Morley *et al.* 1984). CCK-8S has been shown to coexist with neurotensin and dopamine in neurones projecting from the ventral tegmental area to the nucleus accumbens (Seroogy *et al.* 1987), and to a lesser extent in neurones of the substantia nigra projecting to periventricular regions of the caudate (Hokfelt *et al.* 1988).

Evidence suggests that CCK acts as a neurotransmitter in the CNS (for review see Vanderhaegen and Crawley 1985). It is synthesized and stored in nerve terminals and cell bodies; it is released by depolarization; it has specific binding sites; it can affect the firing rate of CNS neurones; and its effects can be interfered with by analogues. Studies have found microiontophoretic application of CCK-8S and CCK-4 on cortical and hippocampal neurones to elicit a strong excitatory action.

CCK receptors are widely distributed throughout the central nervous system with high densities in the striatum and nucleus accumbens (Saito *et al.* 1980; Zarbin *et al.* 1983; Van Dijk *et al.* 1984). Considerable effort has been devoted to characterizing the specificity of brain CCK receptors. So far, two types of CCK receptors have been described: CCK-A receptors which have a higher affinity for sulphated CCK-8 than for de-sulphated CCK-8 (CCK-8US), CCK-4, or gastrin, and CCK-B receptors which have a high affinity for all of these compounds. In the CNS, the majority of CCK receptors belong to the B-type, although CCK-A receptors are found in the area postrema, nucleus tractus solitarius and interpeduncular nucleus, with some interspecies variation (Moran *et al.* 1986; Hill *et al.* 1987*a*; Hill *et al.* 1987*b*).

CHOLECYSTOKININ-TETRAPEPTIDE: A PROVOCATION AGENT FOR RESEARCH IN PANIC DISORDERS?

Guttmacher *et al.* (1983) and Gorman *et al.* (1987) have proposed the following seven criteria for a pharmacological agent to be accepted as an ideal provocative agent. These include, in an order pertinent to research with CCK-4, the following:

1. The agent, in the panicogenic dose, should be safe for routine administration to human subjects.

2. The induced panic attacks should be accompanied by both physical symptoms of panic and subjective symptoms of anxiety, terror, fear, etc.

3. Patients should judge the induced attack to be symptomatically identical or very similar to their regularly occurring spontaneous panic attacks.

4. The induction of panic attacks should be specific to patients with a history of spontaneous panic attacks (absolute specificity); or, the induced attack should occur at a higher rate in these (threshold specificity).

5. The effects of the provocative agent should be consistent in a given patient. If a desensitization effect occurs this should be predictable.

6. Drugs that block spontaneous panic attacks, such as tricyclic anti-depressants, monoamine oxidase inhibitors, or benzodiazepines should also block the pharmacologically-induced attack.

7. Agents that do not block clinical panic attacks should not block the pharmacologically-induced attack.

Any panic-inducing agent which satisfies the above criteria, which is naturally found in the CNS, and which fulfills the criteria for a neurotransmitter could be of theoretical and clinical importance in the study of panic disorders. It is proposed that CCK might be such a provocative agent. The evidence suggesting a role for CCK in the neurobiology of panic and its evaluation with regard to the aforementioned criteria will now be reviewed.

Benzodiazepines are efficacious psychotropics for the treatment of generalized anxiety disorder and are also regarded as an effective mode of treatment in panic disorder (Charney *et al.* 1986; Liebowitz *et al.* 1986). Several researchers have reported the presence of benzodiazepine receptor sites in the CNS (Mohler *et al.* 1978; Braestrup and Squires 1978). Preclinical data suggest that CCK might be implicated in the neurobiology of anxiety. Benzodiazepine receptor agonists selectively antagonize CCK-induced activation of rat CNS neurones (Bradwejn and de Montigny 1984; Bradwejn and de Montigny 1985) and antagonize the effects of CCK in the periphery (Kubota *et al.* 1985). CCK is anxiogenic in animal models of anxiety (Deupree and Hsiao 1987; Csonka *et al.* 1988; Harro *et al.* 1990*a*). Rats with high exploratory activity (non-anxious) in an elevated plus-maze model of anxiety, differ from rats with low exploratory activity (anxious) on CNS CCK and benzodiazepine receptor numbers (Harro *et al.* 1990*b*). CCK antagonists exert an anxiolytic effect in rodent and primate models of anxiety (Hendrie and Dourish 1990; Hughes *et al.* 1990).

Clinical evidence supports the role of CCK in panic disorder. Clinical evidence supports the role of CCK in panic disorder. The effect of CCK-4 was studied in patients with panic disorder (Bradwejn *et al.* 1990). Eleven untreated patients (five women and six men ranging in age from 20 to 51 years) were included in a double-blind study. Each patient received one injection of 2.5 ml of CCK-4 (50 μg in 0.9 M NaCl) and one injection of 2.5 ml of placebo (0.9 M NaCl) on two separate days. All eleven patients panicked following injection of CCK-4, and none following placebo. The CCK-4-induced panic attack included both physical and emotional symptoms, and was described by patients as being phenomenologically identical to their natural panic attacks (criteria 2 and 3), with the exception of a rapid appearance of the symptoms which differed from the more gradual onset of the symptoms during spontaneous attacks. The time until onset of symptoms, after CCK-4 injections was approximately 20 sec. Analysis of symptom profiles experienced during CCK-4-induced panic attacks in 90 patients confirms the reproduction of the symptoms of spontaneous attacks, the unusual rapid appearance of symptoms, and the short time until onset of CCK-4 effect.

De Montigny (1989), in an open uncontrolled study, administered CCK-4 to 10 healthy volunteers at doses ranging from 20 to 100 μg. In seven subjects 'panic-like attacks' were reported to occur. Methodological differences in the de Montigny study and Bradwejn's initial report on panic disorder patients, preclude any comparison of the differential effects of CCK-4 in panic disorder and healthy subjects (criterion 4). A study was recently conducted to determine the specificity of action of CCK-4 (Bradwejn *et al.* 1991). The effect of different doses of CCK was compared in panic disorder patients and healthy volunteers. A double-blind placebo (saline) controlled design with a randomized sequence of injection was used. DSM-III-R criteria, including moderate to severe anxiety, were used to define the occurrence of a panic attack in healthy volunteers. The panic rate with CCK-4 was significantly higher in patients than in healthy volunteers. For example, 25 μg CCK-4 induced a panic attack in 10 of 11 (91 per cent) patients, compared to two of twelve (17 per cent) healthy volunteers. The results support a specificity of action of CCK-4 in panic disorder, as compared to healthy volunteers (criterion 4).

Preliminary findings indicate that the effect of CCK-4 can be reproduced in a test–retest experiment, suggesting that the peptide fulfills criteria 5 (Bradwejn *et al.*, in press).

CONCLUSION

The findings summarized above suggest that CCK might be involved in the neurobiology of panic disorders. Further, CCK satisfies most criteria for an ideal panicogenic agent.

The rapid appearance of symptoms and the short time until onset of panic of 20 sec differs from results obtained with other agents such as lactate. The short time until onset of symptoms after administration of CCK-4 raises questions as to whether the action of the peptide is the result of a direct CNS effect. One explanation for the rapid effects of CCK-4 is that it might act at sites not protected by the blood-brain barrier such as brain–stem nuclei, or at peripheral sites. Hill *et al.* 1988 have demonstrated that the spinal cord dorsal horn of humans and monkeys contains CCK-4 receptors. These receptors can also be found in the area postrema and nucleus tractus solitarius of mammals. These two anatomical locations are thought to be involved in the neurobiology of panic attacks (Gorman *et al.* 1989; Karkanias *et al.* 1989).

Notwithstanding the short time until onset of CCK-4-induced attacks, the profile of symptoms of induced attacks strongly suggests that the peptide reproduces the symptoms of classic panic attacks. The predominant symptom of spontaneous panic attacks has been reported to be marked dyspnea (Klein 1990). Dyspnea has been observed in all panic disorder patients injected with 50 µg of CCK-4 and in 73 per cent of patients injected with 25 µg.

CCK-4 produces panic attacks analogous to another panicogenic agent. Recently, a study was performed which compared the effects of CCK-4 and carbon dioxide in healthy volunteers (Koszycki *et al.* 1991). Subjects received either 25 µg of CCK-4, or a mixture of 35 per cent carbon and 65 per cent oxygen (CO_2). Results for the entire sample revealed that CCK-4 produced more intense symptoms than CO_2. However, the incidence of panic attacks was similar with both substances; 20 per cent (3/14) for CO_2 and 17 per cent (2/12) for CCK-4. Subjects who panicked with either CCK-4 or CO_2 showed no significant differences with respect to the number of symptoms, sum intensity of symptoms, or symptom profile. Using the same methodology, similar results were obtained in panic disorder patients, with the exception that CCK-4 tended to induce a higher incidence of panic attack (Bradwejn and Koszycki, 1991).

The findings reviewed in this chapter support a role for CCK-4 in the neurobiology of panic disorder. At this stage we prefer to view these findings with caution and consider CCK-4 as a potential candidate for a provocation agent which can serve as an additional neurobiological tool. So far, preliminary evidence indicates that CCK-4 fulfills criteria 1 to 5 for an ideal provocation agent. It seems safe (criterion 1), it induces both the physical and emotional symptoms of a panic attack (criterion 2), it induces panic attacks which are identical or very similar to patients' natural panic attacks (criterion 3), it shows a specificity for panic disorder (criterion 4), and its action is predictable (criterion 5). Criteria 6 and 7 remain to be investigated.

ACKNOWLEDGEMENTS

This work was supported by Research Grant MA-10502 from the Medical Research Council of Canada (J. Bradwejn and D. Koszycki).

REFERENCES

Beinfeld, M.C. (1983). Cholecystokinin in the central nervous system: a mini-review. *Neuropeptide*, **3**, 411–27.

Bradwejn, J. and de Montigny, C. (1984). Benzodiazepines antagonize cholecystokinin-induced activation of rat hippocampal neurons. *Nature*, **312**, 363–4.

Bradwejn, J. and de Montigny, C. (1985). Effects of PK 8165, a partial benzodiazepine receptor agonist, on cholecystokinin-induced activation of hippocampal pyramidal neurons: a microiontophoretic study in the rat. *European Journal of Pharmacology*, **112**, 415–18.

Bradwejn, J. and Koszycki, D. (1991). Comparison of the effects of cholecystokinin tetrapeptide and carbon dioxide in panic disorder. *Progress in Neuro-Psychopharmacology and Biological Psychiatry*, **15**, 237–9.

Bradwejn, J., Koszycki, D., and Meterissian, G. (1990). Cholecystokinin-tetrapeptide induced panic attacks in patients with panic disorder. *Canadian Journal of Psychiatry*, **35**, 83–5.

Bradwejn, J., Koszycki, D., and Shriqui, C. (1991). Enhanced sensitivity to cholecystokinin-tetrapeptide in panic disorder. *Archives of General Psychiatry*, 603–610.

Bradwejn, J., Koszycki, D., Payeur, R., Bourin, M., and Borthwick, H. Study of the replication of action of cholecystokinin in panic disorders. *American Journal of Psychiatry*, (in press).

Braestrup, C., and Squires, R.F. (1978). Pharmacological characterization of benzodiazepine receptors in the brain. *European Journal of Pharmacology*, **48**, 263–70.

Charney, D.S., Woods, S.W., Goodman, W.K., Rifkin, B., Kinch, M., Aiken, B. et al. (1986). Drug treatment of panic disorder: the comparative efficacy of imipramine, alprazolam, and trazodone. *Journal of Clinical Psychiatry*, **47**, 580–6.

Csonka, E., Fekete, M., Nagy, G., Szanto-Fekete, M., Feledyg, G., Penke, B., and Kovaks, K. (1988). Anxiogenic effect of cholecystokinin in rats. In *Peptides*, pp. 249–52. Walter de Gruyter, New York.

Deupree, D. and Hsiao, S. (1987). Cholecystokinin octapeptide, proglumide, and conditioned taste avoidance in rats. *Physiological Behaviour*, **41**, 125–8.

Gorman, J.M., Fyer, M.R., Liebowitz, M.R., and Klein, D.F. (1987). In *Psychopharmacology: the third generation of progress* (ed. H.Y. Meltzer). Raven Press, New York.

Gorman, J.M., Liebowitz, M.R., Fyer, A.J., and Stein, J. (1989). Neuro-anatomical hypothesis for panic disorder. *American Journal of Pyschiatry*, **146**, 148–61.

Grant, S.J., and Redmond (Jr), D.E. (1981). In *Psychopharmacology of clonidine* (eds H. Lal and S. Fielding), pp. 5–27. Alan R. Liss, New York.

Guttmacher, L.B., Murphy, D.L., and Insel, T.R. (1983). Pharmacologic models of anxiety. *Comprehensive Psychiatry*, **24**, 312–26.

Harro, J., Pold, M., and Vasar, E. (1990*a*). Anxiogenic-like action of caerulein, a CCK-8 receptor agonist, in the mouse: influence of acute and subchronic diazepam treatment. *Archives of Pharmacology*, **341**, 62–7.

Harro, J., Kiivet, R.A., Lang, A., and Vasar, E. (1990*b*). Rats with anxious or non-anxious type of exploratory behaviour differ in their brain CCK-8 and benzodiazepine receptor characteristics. *Behavioral Brain Research* **39**, 63–71.

Hendrie, C.A. and Dourish, C.T. (1990). Anxiolytic profile of the cholecystokinin antagonist devazepide in mice. *British Journal of Pharmacology*, **99** (suppl.), 138.

Hill, D.R., Shaw, T.M., and Woodruff, G.N. (1987*a*). Species differences in the localization of 'peripheral' type cholecystokinin receptors in rodent brain. *Neuroscience Letters*, **79**, 286–9.

Hill, D.R., Campbell, N.J., Shaw, T.M., and Woodruff, G.N. (1987*b*). Autoradiographic localization and biochemical characterization of peripheral type CCK receptors in rat CNS using highly selective non-peptide CCK agonists. *Journal of Neuroscience*, **7**, 2967–76.

Hill, D.R., Shaw, T.M., and Woodruff, G.N. (1988). Binding sites for 125I-cholecystokinin in primate spinal cord are of the CCK-A subclass. *Neuroscience Letters*, **89**, 133–9.

Hokfelt, T., Herrera-Marschitz, M., Seroogy, K., Ju, G., Staines, W.A., Holets, V. *et al.* (1988). Immunohistochemical studies on cholecystokinin (CCK)-immunoreactive neurons in the rat using sequence specific antisera and with special reference to the caudate nucleus. *Journal of Chemical Neuroanatomy*, **1**, 11–52.

Hughes, J., Boden, P., Costall, B., Domeney, A., Kelly, E., Horwell, D.C. *et al.* (1990). Development of a class of selective cholecystokinin type B receptor antagonists having potent anxiolytic activity. *Proceedings of the National Academy of Sciences (USA)* **87**, 6728–32.

Karkanias, C.D., Block, G.D., Reines, S., and Bradwejn, J. (1989). Neurobiology of panic disorder. Letter. *American Journal of Psychiatry*, **146** (10), 1357.

Klein, D.F. (1990) The physiopathology of spontaneous panic as related to respiratory dyscontrol. *Clinical Neuropharmacology*, **13**, 424–5.

Koszycki, D., Bradwejn, J., and Bourin, M. (1991). Comparison of the effects of cholecystokinin-tetrapeptide and carbon dioxide in healthy volunteers. *European Neuropsychopharmacology*, **1**, 137–42.

Kubota, K., Sugaya, K., Sunagane, N., Matsuoka, Y., and Uruno, T. (1985). Cholecystokinin antagonism by benzodiazepines in the contractile response of the isolated guinea-pig gallbladder. *European Journal of Pharmacology*, **110**, 225–31.

Liebowitz, M.R., Fyer, A.J., Gorman, J.M., Campeas, R., Levin, A., Davies, S.R. *et al.* (1986). Alprazolam in the treatment of panic disorder. *Journal of Clinical Psychopharmacology*, **6**, 13–20.

Maas, J.W., Hattox, S.E., Green, N.M., Landis, D.H. (1977). A direct method for studying 3-methoxy-4-hydroxyphenethyleneglycol (MHPG) by brain in awake animals. *European Journal of Pharmacology*, **46**, 221–28.

Mohler, H., Okada, T., Heiz, P., and Ulrich, J. (1978). Biochemical identification of the site of action of benzodiazepines in human brain by H3-diazepam binding. *Life Sciences*, **22**, 985–96.

de Montigny, C. (1989). Cholecystokinin-tetrapeptide induces panic-like attacks in healthy volunteers. *Archives of General Psychiatry*, **46**, 511–17.

Morley, P.D., Rehfeld, J.F., and Emson, P.C. (1984). Distribution and chromatographic characterization of gastrin and cholecystokinin in the rat central nervous system. *Journal of Neurochemistry*, **42**, 1523–35.

Moran, T.H., Robinson, P.H., Goldrich, M.S., and McHugh, P.R. (1986). Two brain cholecystokinin receptors: implications for behavioral actions. *Brain Research*, **341**, 350–9.

Redmond, D.E., Jr. (1987). Studies of the nucleus locus coeruleus in monkeys and hypothesis for neuropsychopharmacology. In *Psychopharmacology: the third generation of progress*, (ed. H.Y. Meltzer). Raven Press, New York.

Reeve, J.R., Eysselein, V.E., Walsh, J.H., Sankaran, H., Deveney, C.W., Tourtellotte, W.W. *et al.* (1984). Isolation and characterization of biologically active and inactive cholecystokinin-octapeptide from human brain. *Peptides*, **5**, 959–66.

Roberts, G.W., Woodhams, P.L., Polak, J.M., and Crow, T.J. (1982). Distribution of neuropeptides in the limbic system of the rat: the amygdaloid complex. *Neuroscience*, **7**, 99–132.

Saito, A., Sankaran, H., Goldfine, I.D., and Williams, J.A. (1980). Cholecystokinin receptors in the brain: characterization and distribution. *Science*, **208**, 1155–6.

Sauter, A., and Frick, W. (1983). Determination of cholecystokinin tetrapeptide and cholecystokinin octapeptide sulfate in different rat brain regions by high-pressure liquid chromatography with electrochemical detection. *Analytical Biochemistry*, **133**, 307–13.

Seroogy, K.B., Mehta, A., and Fallon, J.H. (1987). Neurotensin and cholecystokinin coexistence within neurons of the ventral mesencephalon: projections to forebrain. *Experimental Brain Research*, **68**, 277–89.

Vanderhaeghen, J.J., and Crawley, J.N. (eds) (1985). Neuronal cholecystokinin. *Annals of the New York Academy of Sciences*, **448**, 198–219.

Van Dijk, A., Richard, J.G., Trzeciak, A., Gillessen, D., and Mohler, H. (1984). Cholecystokinin receptors: biochemical demonstration and autoradiographical localization in rat brain and pancreas using [3H] cholecystokinin as radioligand. *Journal of Neuroscience*, **4**, 1021–33.

Zarbin, M.A., Innis, R.B., Wamsley, J.K., Snyder, S.H., and Kuhar, M.J. (1983). Autoradiographic localization of cholecystokinin receptors in rodent brain. *Journal of Neuroscience*, **3**, 877–906.

10

Changes in biogenic amine neurotransmitters in panic disorder

B.E. LEONARD, J. BUTLER, D. O'ROURKE, and T.J. FAHY

INTRODUCTION

Panic disorder is one of the most prevalent psychiatric disorders, often associated with agoraphobia, with an estimated prevalence of 5–10 per cent (Myers *et al.* 1984). Until recently, the principal biochemical hypothesis advanced to explain the pathological basis of panic disorder implicated a reduction in central gamma-aminobutyric acid (GABA) function (Paul *et al.* 1987) and/or an enhanced central noradrenergic function (Charney *et al.* 1983). The involvement of the GABA-ergic system in the aetiology of anxiety and panic disorder is largely based on the therapeutic efficacy of benzodiazepines in the treatment of various anxiety states; by facilitating central GABA-ergic activity, the benzodiazepines are assumed to reduce central over-arousal which appears to be associated with the clinical features of the illness. Conversely, over-activity of the central noradrenergic system has been shown to produce anxiety and panic symptoms in man and monkeys. Thus, stimulation of the locus coeruleus, an area of which contains the noradrenergic cell bodies, has been shown to initiate anxiety and to raise the concentration of the main central noradrenaline metabolite, 3-methoxy-4-hydroxyphenyl glycol (MHPG) in patients with panic attack; the decrease in plasma MHPG concentrations was found to parallel the response of patients with panic disorder to treatment (Charney *et al.* 1983).

More recently, clinical and experimental evidence has suggested that 5-hydroxytryptamine (serotonin) also plays a role in anxiety (File 1987). Thus, inhibition of the synthesis of this neurotransmitter in the rat brain has been shown to produce the symptoms of anxiety (File and Hyde 1977), while serotonin uptake inhibitors such as zimelidine (Evans *et al.* 1986), clomipramine (Gloger *et al.* 1981) and fluvoxamine (Den Boer *et al.* 1987) have been found to reduce the incidence of panic attacks in patients. The infusion of lactate consistently initiates panic attack in patients suffering from panic disorder. While the precise mechanism whereby lactate infusion causes panic symptoms is uncertain, Lingjaerde (1985) has shown that lactate will facilitate the transport of serotonin into the platelets of patients with this disorder and has speculated that, as a consequence, the inter-synaptic concentration of the amine is reduced which, in the brain, might lead to a reduction in the inhibitory effect of serotonin on the firing of the locus coeruleus. The attraction of this hypothesis lies in its ability to explain the beneficial effects of serotonin uptake inhibitors in the treatment of panic disorder; by reducing serotonin uptake centrally, drugs such as clomipramine and imipramine facilitate serotonergic function and thereby reduce the symptoms of the illness. The β-adrenoceptor agonist isoprenaline has been shown to produce qualitatively similar effects to lactate (Yeragani *et al.* 1988), which lends further support to the view that an imbalance between the noradrenergic and serotonergic systems are crucially involved in the symptoms of panic attack.

The purpose of this chapter will be to consider the pharmacological and biochemical evidence that implicates a disorder of the noradrenergic and serotonergic systems in panic disorder.

PHARMACOLOGICAL EVIDENCE: EFFICACY OF ANTIDEPRESSANTS IN TREATING THE SYMPTOMS OF PANIC DISORDER

Sargant and his colleagues were the first to suggest that the monoamine oxidase inhibitors (MAOIs) were effective in 'atypical depression' (Sargant and Dally 1962; Sargant 1961). Such patients had symptoms of both somatic and psychic anxiety, hypochondriasis, phobias, and hysteria; depression was also often associated with the symptoms. Kelly *et al.* (1970) later showed that panic attacks were often associated with 'atypical depression' and, in a retrospective study of over 200 patients, suggested that the MAOIs might have potent anti-panic and anti-phobic activity. Of the non-selective MAOIs that have been studied in the treatment of panic disorder, phenelzine would appear to produce a consistent beneficial response. In their detailed studies in which phenelzine was compared with imipramine and placebo, Sheehan *et al.* (1980; 1987), phenelzine was shown to be consistently superior to imipramine, both drugs being superior to placebo. Tyrer and Shawcross (1988), in their review of the use of MAOIs in the treatment of anxiety disorder, concluded that the MAOIs are somewhat more effective than tricyclic antidepressants in the treatment of anxiety disorders and when phobic anxiety is an important component of a depressive disorder. This view concurs with that of Liebowitz *et al.* (1988) who compared 10 major double-blind control trials of various antidepressants in the treatment of panic disorder.

Kahn *et al.* (1987) studied the effects of clomipramine and 5-hydroxytryptophan (5-HTP) in a double-blind placebo controlled trial in a group of 45 patients with anxiety disorders, and found that clomipramine was highly effective while 5-HTP was moderately effective in attenuating the symptoms; clomipramine was shown to be effective in reducing the depressive as well as the anxiety symptoms, while 5-HTP had little effect on the depressive symptoms. It should be emphasized that although clomipramine is a potent serotonin uptake inhibitor, its major metabolite desmethyl clomipramine inhibits specifically noradrenaline uptake (Carlsson *et al.* 1969). The specific serotonin uptake inhibitor, zimeldine, was shown to be superior to imipramine in reducing the symptoms of agoraphobia and panic attack (Evans *et al.* 1986). Kahn *et al.* (1986), in a double-blind placebo-controlled study of imipramine, chlordiazepoxide, and placebo, showed that the tricyclic antidepressant was superior to placebo and chlordiazepoxide. Such findings suggest that both serotonin and noradrenaline are probably involved both in the aetiology of panic disorder and in the therapeutic effect of the antidepressants.

The highly specific serotonin uptake inhibitor, fluvoxamine, has been shown to be equi-effective with clomipramine in attenuating the symptoms of agoraphobia and panic attack (Den Boer *et al.* 1987), which adds support to the hypothesis that an abnormality in the central serotonergic system is implicated in the pathophysiology of agoraphobia and panic disorder. However, it should be noted that the anti-panic effect of the triazolobenzodiazepine alprazolam does not appear to be mediated by changes in the serotonergic system. Thus, Charney and Henninger (1986) reported that the ability of tryptophan to increase prolactin secretion did not differ between patients with panic attack and healthy controls; the prolactin response was unaltered by alprazolam treatment even though the drug was shown to have a beneficial therapeutic effect.

CHANGES IN NEUROTRANSMITTERS ASSOCIATED WITH PANIC DISORDER

Neurotransmitter changes associated with panic disorder

The role of serotonin in the aetiology of anxiety was first suggested by Wise and co-workers (1982), following their studies in which the anxiolytic effects of benzodiazepines in rodents could be counteracted by the intraventricular administration of serotonin. Following such studies, it was postulated that the benzodiazepines reduced the functional activity of serotonin in the brain. Clinical evidence implicating a disorder of the serotonergic system in panic attack has been provided by the studies of Kahn and Van Praag (1988) and Charney *et al.* (1987). In these studies, the selective serotonin agonist *m*-chlorophenyl piperazine (*m*CPP) was found to induce anxiety and panic attacks in patients with panic disorder, but not in control subjects; *m*CPP also induced a significant release of cortisol in the patients with panic disorder but not in the controls or in depressed patients. These authors conclude that the serotonin receptors are hypersensitive in patients with panic disorder, which provides a rational basis for the use of drugs like the benzodiazepines that either reduce the turnover of serotonin, presumably by facilitating inhibitory neurotransmission and thus reducing serotonin release, or reduce the turnover of serotonin by impeding the uptake mechanism (e.g. the selective serotonin uptake inhibitors such as clomipramine, fluoxetine, and fluvoxamine).

Human platelets

Another experimental approach that has been used to investigate changes in the serotonergic system in patients with panic disorder, relies on the fact that human platelets have many functional properties that are similar to the nerve terminal. Thus the platelet membrane has a high affinity, energy-dependent, and Na^+-dependent uptake system for serotonin that is physiologically and pharmacologically similar to that found on nerve terminals in the brain. Furthermore, there are receptors on the platelet membrane that selectively respond to serotonin and noradrenaline; these receptors appear to be of the $5\text{-}HT_2$ type (Leysen *et al.* 1983) and α_2-adrenoceptor type (Cameron *et al.* 1984). On stimulation these receptors cause aggregation of the platelets.

McIntyre and co-workers (1989) reported that the uptake of serotonin was significantly higher in untreated patients with panic attack, while the serotonin content of the platelets was found to be unchanged when compared to control subjects. This confirmed the earlier findings of these investigators (Norman *et al.* 1986) and others (Balon *et al.* 1987). However, in a recently completed study of 60 patients with panic disorder, we have shown that the uptake of serotonin was significantly reduced in the patients before the commencement of treatment, and did not completely normalize following 6 weeks treatment with lofepramine, clomipramine, or placebo. The reason for the discrepancy between our findings and those of these investigators is unclear.

Another experimental approach which has been used to assess changes in serotonergic function in panic disorder has involved measurement of the [^{3}H]-imipramine binding sites on the platelet membrane. The imipramine binding site is postulated to modulate the transport of sero-tonin into the platelet or nerve ending, and while initial studies suggested that the density of these sites was reduced in platelets from depressed patients, more recent studies have failed to confirm such evidence. In patients with panic disorder, Lewis *et al.* (1985) and Marazziti (1989) found evidence to suggest that the imipramine binding sites were reduced in agorophobia patients, although other investigators could not find any difference between the density of these binding sites in such patients and control subjects (Pecknold and Suranyi-Cadotte 1986; Nutt and Fraser 1987; Schneider *et al.* 1987). It would therefore appear that, as in endogenous depression, there is little convincing evidence to suggest that the imipramine binding site is altered in patients with panic disorder with, or without, associated agoraphobia.

Role of the sympathetic system

Despite the ample circumstantial evidence indicating an over-activity of the central sympathetic system which has already been discussed, direct evidence to verify such a hypothesis is limited. Thus Schneider *et al.* (1987) reported that the plasma noradrenaline and adrenaline concentrations were unchanged in a group of 8 patients with panic attack and agoraphobia when compared with control subjects, while Nutt and Frazer (1987) found that the platelet α_2-adrenoceptor density was unchanged in a group of 15 patients with panic disorder. There findings conflict with those of Butler *et al.* (1985) who, in a preliminary study of the changes in α- and β-adrenoceptor function and density on platelets and lymphocytes from a group of 14 patients with panic disorder, found that the densities of both α_2- and β-adrenoceptors were increased, as was the functional activity of the α-adrenoceptors on the platelet membrane as assessed by the noradrenaline elicited aggregation response. To further complicate the picture, Brown *et al.* (1988) reported that the density of lymphocyte β-adrenoceptors was decreased in a group of 17 patients with panic attack associated with agoraphobia. Again, the reason for the disparity in the biochemical data is unclear as similar diagnostic procedures were used in all studies to classify the patients.

Changes in peripheral markers of serotonergic and adrenergic function in patients with panic attack and following treatment with placebo clomipramine or lofepramine

The authors have recently completed a study of 66 patients with panic disorder, fulfilling the DSM-III criteria for panic attack, together with a group of age and sex matched controls. The purpose of this study was to assess their noradrenergic and serotonergic status (using the platelet and lymphocyte as peripheral markers of central monoamine function), before the commencement of treatment and following a 10 day 'wash-out' period.

The patients were randomly assigned to one of three treatment groups (a) placebo, (b) clomipramine, and (c) lofepramine on a double-blind basis. All patients received weekly behavioural therapy throughout the initial 6 weeks of the drug or placebo treatment. At the end of the 6-week period, the behavioural therapy ceased and those patients in the placebo group were randomly allocated to the clomipramine or lofepramine treatment groups. Treatment was then continued for a total period of 6 months, the dose of the medication being tapered down slowly from the 12th week of treatment so that the patients were drug free at the end of the study. In addition to the Hamilton Anxiety and Depression scores, the Wakefield Depression scores and the Montgomery and Asberg Depression scores, all patients were assessed by the Clinical Global Impression and Panic Attack Frequency scores periodically throughout the 6 months of the study. Blood samples were taken at the commencement of the study (W0) and at the end of Weeks 1, 2, 4, 6, 8, 12, and 24. The methods used to assess serotonergic and noradrenergic function on platelets and lymphocytes have been summarized elsewhere (Butler *et al.* 1988). A detailed publication of this study is in preparation and therefore only an overview of the findings will be presented for the first 6-week period of treatment (Fahy *et al.*, in press, Butler *et al.*, in press).

In an attempt to determine whether correlations existed between the clinical response to treatment and any of the biochemical parameters, a marked improvement as assessed by the Clinical Global Impression and Panic Attack Frequency scores, and a reduction in the Hamilton Anxiety Score to <5, was taken to be evidence of treatment response.

Table 10.1 gives an indication of the response of patients to treatment at the end of the initial 6-week period of the study.

It is evident that all three groups improved and that there was a marginal benefit in the two antidepressant groups over the placebo group. Of the antidepressants, lofepramine appeared to be better tolerated by the patients.

Table 10.2 gives an overview of the changes in the markers of serotonergic and noradrenergic function in patients with panic attack before and following 6-week treatment with placebo, clomipramine, or lofepramine. It should be emphasized that these results are for those patients showing the most severe symptoms before the commencement of treatment compared to those showing a complete response to treatment at the end of 6 weeks. In the detailed account of this study to be published, the biochemical changes associated with panic symptoms of moderate, mild, or borderline severity will also be presented (Fahy *et al.*, in press). Scrutiny of all the data however, shows a qualitative similarity with those

TABLE 10.1. *Effect of placebo or antidepressant treatment on patients with panic attack*

Treatment group			
Outcome	Placebo (N = 23)	Clomipramine (N = 16)	Lofepramine (N = 23)
Clinical Global Impression scale			
No change	5 (22%)	1 (6%)	1 (4%)
Better	17 (74%)	15 (94%)	21 (91%)
Worse	1 (4%)	0	1 (4%)
Panic Attack Frequency scale			
	(N = 24)	(N = 18)	(N = 24)
No change	7 (29%)	4 (22%)	2 (8%)
Better	16 (67%)	14 (78%)	22 (92%)
Worse	1 (4%)	0	0

presented here. In summary, it would appear that the noradrenaline-induced platelet aggregation is slightly enhanced, and that the number of α_2-receptors on the platelet membrane is increased, in untreated patients, and that both are unchanged following placebo or antidepressant treatment.

The number of β-adrenoceptors on the lymphocyte membrane is also increased and remains elevated at the end of the treatment period. Thus, there is evidence that the sympathetic system is hyperactive in the patients and remains unchanged despite their apparent response to treatment. It should be noted that these parameters remain elevated even following 6 months of drug treatment!

The results shown in Table 10.2 also demonstrate that the serotonergic system is abnormal in patients with panic attack, and remain largely unchanged despite the complete normalization of the patients behaviour following drug treatment. Thus, serotonin-induced aggregation, an index of 5-HT$_2$ receptor responsiveness, is reduced and the number of 5-HT$_2$ receptors on the platelet membrane is elevated in the untreated patients and does not change appreciably following effective treatment. These results suggest that the coupling between the receptor and the secondary messenger unit on the inner platelet membrane is defective in panic patients. A similar change has been found in patients with endogenous depression (Healy *et al*. 1985). The transport of ^{3}H-5-HT also appears to be slightly defective in panic patients, but this abnormality would not seem to be as pronounced as that found in patients suffering from endogenous depression (Healy *et al*. 1985).

TABLE 10.2. *Parameters of noradrenergic and serotonergic function in panic patients before (W0) and following (W6) treatment with placebo, clomipramine, or lofepramine*

		Control	Placebo	Clomipramine	Lofepramine
NA aggregation					
% ADP	W0	17.02±0.83	26.66±3.42 ($N = 9$)	199.66±4.37 ($N = 3$)	32.14±7.20 ($N = 7$)*
	W6	($N = 45$)	23.00±3.62 ($N = 4$)	22.25±2.75 ($N = 8$)	16.91±2.28 ($N = 12$)
5-HT aggregation					
% ADP	W0	34.30±1.25	17.87±4.86 ($N = 8$)***	10.66±0.88 ($N = 3$)***	17.50±4.02 ($N = 6$)***
	W6	($N = 42$)	17.40±4.00 ($N = 5$)***	28.75±4.99 ($N = 8$)	10.66±2.94 ($N = 12$)***
5-HT V_{max}	W0	188.37±62.68	169.88±62.7 ($N = 9$)	98.33±63.8 ($N = 3$)	131.4±30.1 ($N = 8$)
	W6	($N = 51$)	209.00±83.0 ($N = 4$)	166.6±24.9 ($N = 9$)	167.0±2.97 ($N = 10$)
5-HT K_m	W0	0.56±0.66	0.59±0.18 ($N = 9$)	0.17±0.07 ($N = 3$)*	0.58±0.23 ($N = 8$)
	W6	($N = 51$)	0.33±0.09 ($N = 4$)*	0.69±0.14 ($N = 9$)	0.95±0.28 ($N = 10$)
(^{3}H)-Ketanserin					
(5-HT$_2$) B_{max}	W0	20.0±0.46	34.0±4.23 ($N = 10$)***	39.33±0.88 ($N = 3$)***	32.25±3.64 ($N = 8$)***
	W6	($N = 53$)	31.20±3.13 ($N = 5$)***	27.88±3.18 ($N = 9$)**	35.81±2.65 ($N = 11$)***
(^{3}H)-Rauwolcine					
($\alpha 2$) B_{max}	W0	124.9±1.87	201.9±20.6 ($N = 6$)***	155.0±45.9 ($N = 3$)	201.3±19.3 ($N = 8$)***
	W6	($N = 53$)	143.3±25.9 ($N = 4$)	151.9±17.6 ($N = 9$)	186.5±27.6 ($N = 11$)*
(^{3}H)-DHA					
(β) β_{max}	W0	5.68±1.07	9.66±1.07 ($N = 9$)*	9.00±2.52 ($N = 3$)	11.88±1.16 ($N = 8$)***
	W6	($N = 53$)	7.75±1.79 ($N = 4$)	7.33±1.01 ($N = 9$)	8.88±0.92 ($N = 9$)*

The results shown express only those patients who exhibited severe symptoms at week 0, as assessed by the Clinical Global Impression score, and a total absence of symptoms at week 6 of treatment. In this way an indication of the relationship between the maximal clinical response to treatment and the biochemical parameters measured could be assessed. * $p < 0.05$; ** $p < 0.005$; *** $p´ < 0.001$ vs control (2-tailed t-test).

Thus, this study provides evidence for a change in peripheral markers of both noradrenergic and serotonergic activity which do not alter with response of the patient to effective treatment. Furthermore, these abnormalities persist for at least 6 months of active drug treatment. It may be concluded that these parameters are trait markers of panic attack.

CONCLUSION

Table 10.3 summarizes the results of the various studies in which peripheral markers of serotonergic and noradrenergic function have been determined in patients with panic disorder. While no unequivocal changes in these parameters in panic disorder are apparent, the results do lend some support to the hypothesis that these two neurotransmitter systems may be associated with the psychopathology of panic disorder. Furthermore, the clinical and biochemical overlap between panic disorder and endogenous depression, as indicated by the responsiveness of both conditions to antidepressant treatment, and the changes in the peripheral markers of central and serotonergic function (Healy *et al.* 1985), lend credibility to the view that panic attack is part of the spectrum of major affective disorder and possibly distinct from generalized anxiety disorder. Other investigators have produced clinical and biochemical evidence in support of this view (Uhde *et al.* 1985).

The recognition of the relatively high frequency of panic disorder in the general population in recent years has led to a widespread interest in the condition by biological psychiatrists. This has been instrumental in the development of more specific drug therapies to treat the major symptoms of the disorder, and has also led to an attempt to define the underlying pathology of the condition by assessing the changes in platelet and lymphocyte markers that occur concomitantly with the symptoms. While there is good evidence to suggest that the noradrenergic, serotonergic, and possibly the GABA-ergic systems are causally linked to the symptoms of the illness, there is an urgent need to undertake detailed longitudinal studies on a substantial number of patients to adequately test the hypothesis that such neurotransmitters are responsible for the psychopathology of the disorder.

ACKNOWLEDGEMENT

The authors are grateful to the Pharmacia-Leo Co., of Helsingborg, Sweden for financial support and to the Health Research Board of Ireland, for financial support.

TABLE 10.3. *Summary of the changes in the activities of noradrenergic and serotonergic systems in panic disorder*

Biochemical parameter	Number of patients in study	Change reported	Reference
1. β-receptor density on lymphocytes	21	Decreased β_{max}	Brown *et al.* 1988
2. "	14	Increased β_{max}	Butler *et al.* 1988
3. 2 receptor density	15	Unchanged β_{max}	Nutt and Frazer 1987
4. "	14	Increased β_{max}	Butler *et al.* 1988
5. Noradrenaline induced platelet aggregation	14	Increased response	Butler *et al.* 1988
6. Plasma adrenaline and noradrenaline concentrations	8	Unchanged	Shneider *et al.* 1987
7. [^{3}H]-5-HT uptake into platelets	17	Increased uptake (V_{max})	McIntyre *et al.* 1989
8. " "	45	Increased uptake (V_{max})	Norman *et al.* 1986
9. " "	14	Decreased uptake (V_{max})	Butler *et al.* 1988
10. Serotonin-induced	14	Decreased response platelet aggregation	Butler *et al.* 1988
11. Platelet serotonin content	18	Unchanged	Balon *et al.* 1987
12. [^{3}H]-imipramine binding	9	Slight decrease in B_{max}	Marazziti 1989
13. " "	?	Decrease in β_{max}	Lewis *et al.* 1985
14. " "	15	Unchanged β_{max}	Nutt and Frazer 1987

REFERENCES

Balon, R., Pohl, R., Veragani, V., Rainey, D.H., and Oxenkrug, G. (1987). Platelet serotonin levels in panic disorder. *Acta Psychiatrica Scandinavica*, **75**, 315–17.

Brown, S.L., Charney, D.S., Woods, S.W., Henninger, G.R., and Tallman, J. (1988). Lymphocyte β-adrenergic receptor binding in panic disorder. *Psychopharmacology*, **94**, 24–8.

Butler, J., Tannion, M., O'Rourke, D., Fahy, T.J., and Leonard, B.E. (1985). Functional changes in the adrenergic and serotonergic systems in patients with panic disorder. In *Progress in catecholamine research part C: Clinical aspects*, pp. 399–407. Alan Liss, New York.

Butler, J., Tannian, M., O'Rourke, D., Fahy, T.J., and Leonard, B.E. (1988). Change in biogenic amines in panic disorder. In *Progress in catecholamine research* (ed. R.H. Belmaker, M. Sandler, and A. Dahlstrom), pp. 399–407. Liss, New York.

Butler, J., O'Halloran, A., and Leonard, B.E. (1992). The Galway Study of Panic Disorder II: Changes in some peripheral markers of noradrenergic and serotonergic function in DSMIIIR Panic Disorder. *Journal of Affective Disorders*, (in press).

Cameron, O.G., Smith, C.B., Hollingsworth, P.J., Neese, R.M., and Curtis, G.C. (1984). Platelet alpha-2 adrenergic receptor binding and plasma catecholamines: before and during imipramine treatment in patients with panic anxiety. *Archives of General Psychiatry*, **41**: 1144–8.

Carlsson, A., Corrodi, H., Fuxe, K., and Hokfelt, J. (1969). Effect of antidepressant drugs on the depletion of intraneuronal brain 5-hydroxytryptamine stores caused by 4 methyl-ethyl metatyramine. *European Journal of Pharmacology*, **5**, 537–66.

Charney, D.S., Henninger, G.R., and Redmond, J.R. (1983). Yohimbine induced anxiety and increased noradrenergic function in humans: effects of diazepam and clonidine. *Life Sciences*, **33**, 9–29.

Charney, D.S. and Heninger, G.R. (1986). Serotonin function in panic disorders. *Archives of General Psychiatry*, **43**, 1059–65.

Charney, D.S., Woods, S.W., Goodman, W.K., and Heninger, G.R. (1987). Serotonin function in anxiety. II. Effects of the serotonin agonist *m*CPP in panic disorder patients and healthy subjects. *Psychopharmacology* **92**, 14–24.

Den Boer, J.A., Westenberg, H.G.M., Kamerbeck, W.D.J., Verhoeven, W.M.A., and Kahn, R.S. (1987). Effect of serotonin uptake inhibitors in anxiety disorders: a double-blind comparison of clomipramine and fluvoxamine. *International Journal of Clinical Psychopharmacology*, **2**, 21–32.

Evans, L., Kenardy, J., Schneiderm, P., and Hoey, H. (1986). Effect of a selective serotonin uptake inhibitor in agorophobia with panic attacks. A double blind comparison of zimelidine, imipramine and placebo. *Acta Psychiatrica Scandinavica*, **73**, 49–53.

Fahy, T.J., O'Rourke, D., Brophy, J., Schatzmann, W., and Sciascia, S. (1992). The Galway study of panic disorder. I: Clomipramine and Lofepramine in DSMIIIR Panic Disorder: a placebo controlled trial. *Journal of Affective Disorders*, (in press).

File, S.F. and Hyde, J. (1977). The effects of 1-chlorophenylalanine and ethanolamine-O-sulphate in an animal test of anxiety. *Journal of Pharmacy and Pharmacology* **29**, 735–38.

File, S.F. (1987). The neurochemistry of anxiety. In *Anti-anxiety agents* (eds G.D. Burrows, T.R. Niorman, and B. Davies, pp. 13–34. Elsevier, Amsterdam.

Gloger, S., Grundhaus, L., Birmacher, B., and Troudart, J. (1981). Treatment of spontaneous panic attacks with clomipramine. *American Journal Psychiatry* **138**, 1215–17.

Healy, D., Carney, P.A., O'Halloran, A., and Leonard, B.E. (1985). Peripheral adrenoceptors and serotonin receptors in depression: changes associated with response to treatment with trazodone and amitriptyline. *Journal of Affective Disorders*, **9**, 285–96.

Kahn, R.J., McNair, D.M., Kipman, R.S., Covi, L., Rickels, K., Downing, R. *et al.* (1986). Imipramine and chlordiazepoxide in depressive and anxiety disorders. III Efficacy in anxious out-patients. *Archives of General Psychiatry*, **43**, 1059–65.

Kahn, R.S., Westengberg, H.G.M., Verhoeven, W.M.A., Gispen-de Wied, C.C., and Kamerbeek, W.D.J. (1987). Effect of a serotonin precursor and uptake inhibitor in anxiety disorders: a double-blind comparison of 5-hydroxytryptophan, clomipramine and placebo. *International Journal of Clinical Psychopharmacology* **2**, 33–45.

Kahn, R.S. and Van Praag, H.M. (1988). A serotonin hypothesis of panic disorder. *Human Psychopharmacology*, **3**, 285–8.

Kelly, D., Guirguis, W., Frommer, E., Mitchell-Heggs, N., and Sargant, W. (1970). Treatment of phobic states with antidepressants: a retrospective study of 246 patients. *British Journal of Psychiatry*, **116**, 387–98.

Lewis, D.A., Noyes, R., Goryell, W., and Clancy, J. (1985). Tritiated imipramine binding to platelets is decreased in patients with agorabphobia. *Psychiatry Research*, **16**, 1–9.

Leysen, J.E., Gommeren, W., and De Clerck, F. (1983). Demonstration of S-2 receptor binding sites on cat blood platelets using [^{3}H]-ketanserin. *European Journal of Pharmacology*, **88**, 125–30.

Liebowitz, M.R., Fyer, A.J., Gorman, J.M., Campeas, R.B., Sandberg, D.P.H. Hollander, E. *et al.* (1988). Tricyclic therapy of the DSM III anxiety disorders: a review of the implications for further research. *Journal of Psychiatric Research*, **22** (Suppl. 1), 7–31.

Lingjaerde, O. (1985). Lactate-induced panic attacks: possible involvement of serotonin reuptake stimulation. *Acta Psychiatrica Scandinavica*, **72**, 206–8.

McIntyre, I.M., Judd, F.K., Burrows, G.D., and Norman, T.R. (1989). Serotonin in panic disorder: platelet uptake and concentration. *International Journal of Clininical Psychopharmacology*, **4**, 1–6.

Marazziti, D. (1989). Imipramine binding in panic disorder. *Pharmacopsychiatry*, **2**, 128–9.

Myers, T.K., Weissman, M.M., Tischler, G.L., Holzer, C.E., and Leaf, Ph.J. (1984). Six month prevalence of psychiatric disorders in three communities 1980–1982. *Archives of General Psychiatry*, **41**, 959–67.

Norman, J.R., Judd, F.K., Gregory, M., James, R.H., Kimber, N.M., McIntyre, I.M., and Burrows, G.D. (1986). Platelet serotonin uptake in panic disorder. *Journal of Affective Disorders*, **11**, 69–72.

Nutt, D.J. and Frazer, S. (1987). Platelet binding studies in panic disorder. *Journal of Affective Disorders*, **12**, 7–11.

Paul, S.M., Marangos, P.J., and Skolnick, P. (1987). The benzodiazepine-GABA chloride ionophore receptor complex: common site of minor tranquillizer action. *Biological Psychiatry*, **16**, 213–29.

Pecknold, J.C. and Suranyi-Cadotte, B.E. (1986). Panic disorder and depression: serotonin uptake with [^{3}H]-imipramine studies. *Clinical Neuropharmacology*, **9** (Suppl. 4), 46–8.

Sargant, W. (1961). Drugs in the treatment of depression. *British Medical Journal*, **1**, 25–7.

Sargant, W. and Dally, P. (1962). Treatment of anxiety states by antidepressant drugs. *British Medical Journal*, **1**, 6–9.

Schneider, P., Evans, L., Ross-Lee, L., Wiltshire, B., Eadie, M., Kennedy, J., and Joey, H. (1987). Plasma biogenic amine levels in agoraphobia with panic attacks. *Pharmacopsychiatry*, **20**, 102–4.

Sheehan, D.V., Ballenger, J., and Jacobsen, G. (1980). Treatment of endogenous anxiety with phobic, hysterical and hypochondriacal symptoms. *Archives of General Psychiatry*, **37**, 51–9.

Sheehan, D.V., Ballenger, J., and Jacobsen, G. (1987). Relative efficacy of monoamine oxidase inhibitors and tricyclic antidepressants in the treatment of endogenous anxiety. In *Anxiety: new research and changing concepts*. (eds D.F. Klein and J. Rabkin), pp. 47–67. Raven Press, New York.

Tyrer, P. and Shawcross, C. (1988). Monoamine oxidase inhibitors in anxiety disorders. *Journal of Psychiatric Research*, **22** (Suppl. 1), 87–98.

Uhde, T.W., Boulenger, J.-P., Roy-Byrne, P.P., Graci, M.F., Vitton, B.J., and Post, R.M. (1985). Longitudinal course of panic disorder: clinical and biological considerations. *Progress in Neuro-Psychopharmacology and Biolical Psychiatry*, **9**, 39–51.

Stein, L. (1980). Behavioral neurochemistry of benzodiazepines. *Arzneimittel-forschung*, **30**, (**5a**), 868–73.

Yeragani, V.K., Rainey, J.M., Pohl, R., Balon, R., Berchou, R., Jolly, S., and Lycaki, H. (1988). Preinfusion anxiety and laboratory induced panic attacks in panic disorder patients. *Journal of Clinical Psychiatry*, **49**, 302–6.

11

A psychobiological model for panic: including models for the mechanisms involved in the regulation of mood and anxiety and implications for behavioural and pharmacological therapies

G.W. ASHCROFT, L.G. WALKER, and A. LYLE

INTRODUCTION

Whilst the main thrust of this chapter will be towards providing a model for both the psychological and pharmacological treatment of panic attacks, the model will also be extended to include the brain mechanisms involved in the regulation of human mood (affect) and anxiety.

The basis for the discussion of these models is the presence in the brain of mechanisms which provide the neural substrates for the behavioural and feeling states we recognize as anxiety and mood. Depression, elation, fear and, in some situations, panic are normal reactions to appropriate environmental stimuli. However, each of these reactions can also occur in less appropriate circumstances and provide less adaptive responses when they may become classified as 'illness'.

From a biological standpoint, panic attacks are seen as a reaction to the threatened failure of secure exploration, when escape from a threatening situation is perceived as impossible. Panic thus differs from anticipatory anxiety in that it involves an abrupt suspension of ongoing behaviours. Panic attacks are therefore the equivalent of freeze reactions in animals and may increase the chance of survival in the absence of a more adaptive alternative by drawing less attention to the animal. It is interesting that many patients experiencing a panic attack in a large store will freeze rather than run, giving their reason as 'not wanting to draw attention' to themselves.

Of course, in many situations panic occurs with minimal threat or even in the absence of immediate threat — so-called 'spontaneous attacks'. To explain this phenomenon we need to include the concept of a variable threshold for the triggering of panic, and much of the authors' clinical effort is directed towards assessing the physical and psychological variables which alter the triggering threshold. Examples of these influences include changes in the social environment involving supportive attachments or bereavement. Separation or threat of loss increase vulnerability to the development of panic attacks. Internal events which alter the threshold include, for example, the onset of a depressive illness and a range of endocrine and metabolic changes such as hyperventilation-induced changes in pCO_2.

Interacting with these factors which act to modify the threshold of the trigger mechanism will be changes in the intensity of precipitating stimuli. Here it is the perceived significance of the stimulus that is important. Physiological components of the panic response, for example tachycardia, may become incorporated into the perception of threat and themselves contribute to the culmination of the panic.

The authors have not found the American DSM-III-R concept of panic disorder to be a useful one. Rather, an attempt is made in this chapter to understand the occurrence of the attacks in the context in which they are occurring, and to evaluate the importance of the different factors which may have changed the threshold or increased the perceived intensity of the attacks.

The chapter begins by reviewing animal studies which may have a bearing on the mechanisms of panic, anxiety, and mood. Following a brief presentation of the model, its application to drug therapy and to psychological treatments is then discussed. Thereafter, an outline of its use in the choice of treatment for particular patients is provided, including the option of combined drug/psychological treatment.

THE MODEL (Fig. 11.1)

Exploration

The authors' clinical studies in depression, hypomania, anxiety, and panic have led them to propose the central importance of brain mechanisms in the mediation and regulation of exploratory behaviours (Ashcroft 1972; Ashcroft 1973; Ashcroft *et al.* 1987).

Exploration comprises a complex behavioural pattern involved in searching for familiar stimuli and attending to novel stimuli. Its implementation facilitates the achievement of primary drive satisfaction and allows maximum exploitation of the environment.

In this model the subjective elements of mood states are seen as the labelling of the current direction and intensity of exploratory drive; hence

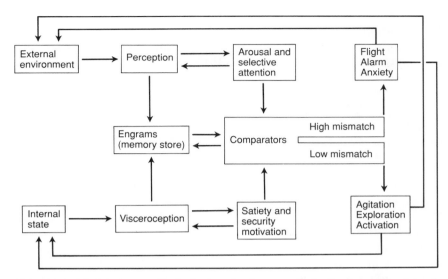

FIG. 11.1. Model for psychological and pharmacological treatment of panic attacks.

reduced exploration will normally result in depressed feelings and increased exploration in elevation of mood.

Relevance of animal studies to the understanding of human mood and anxiety

Exploratory systems

Makanjuola *et al.* (1977*a*, 1977*b*, 1980, 1992) investigated the role of dopaminegic systems in the mediation of exploratory, locomotor, and stereotyped behaviours in the rat. Selective bilateral destruction of dopaminergic nerve terminals in the accumbens nuclei by stereotactic injection of 6-hydroxydopamine reduced locomotor and exploratory behaviour. Bilateral injections of dopamine into the nucleus accumbens of nialamide pretreated rats produced stimulation of exploration. Similar injections into the caudate-putamen produced intense stereotyped behaviour. These results suggest that the nucleus accumbens is on the efferent pathway for mediation of exploratory responses.

Costall *et al.* (1982) have shown that cycles of increased exploratory activity are produced in the rat following chronic (13-day) infusions of dopamine into the dominant amygdalae.

Makanjuola *et al.* (1992) have recently produced evidence that the ventral pallidum lies on the efferent pathway for the mediation of exploration, and includes a GABAminergic synapse in this part of the pathway.

The hippocampal comparator

Gray (1982) suggested that systems in the hippocampus function as a comparator recognizing and responding to novelty and assessing its significance in terms of previous experience. Mason and Fibiger (1979) conclude that the dorsal noradrenergic bundle (DNAB) functions to determine selective attention to relevant stimuli in the environment. Combining both these observations, we can suggest that input from the DNAB into the comparator will alter the sensitivity to novelty perhaps by changing the signal-to-noise ratio in the system.

Behaviour in strange and familiar environments —
regulation of the response to novelty

Ellison (1975) studied in rats the effects of selective lesions of brain 5-hydroxytryptamine (5-HT)and noradrenergic (NA) systems on exploration in novel and familiar environments. In the open-field test (strange environment), low 5-HT rats showed evidence of fear and were inhibited in exploration while low NA rats 'fearlessly ambulated about the enclosure'. In the familiar colony environment this pattern was reversed, with the low 5-HT rats appearing fearless while low NA rats failed to explore, spending most of the time in their burrows.

Neuronal substrate for behavioural systems outlined in Fig. 11.1 — a model

The comparator systems are in the temporal lobe, receiving information regarding external and internal environments via the sensory systems and evaluating this in terms of previous experience. The sensitivity of the comparators to novelty is influenced by inputs from noradrenergic and 5-HT systems, increased input from the former increasing the impact of novelty, and increase in 5-HT input decreasing the sensitivity to novelty. In this way the result of the Ellison experiments can be explained for the 5-HT lesions: they will increase activity in the low novelty home environment, whilst in the open field the degree of novelty will be so high as to produce an aversive response.

Efferent systems are those by which positive and negative behaviours (e.g. approach, exploration, flight, and in man the accompanying feeling states of elation, depression, fear, and anxiety) are mediated.

The negative system (limbic system) has received much attention. Less attention has been given to the exploratory systems which involve temporal lobe (amygdala), nucleus accumbens, and ventral pallidum. We suggest here that altered activity in this system mediates the exploratory responses to novelty and, in man, the affective responses of depression and elation.

Panic attacks and the system

As has already been suggested, panic provides an alternative response under threat to 'flight or fight'. It is an all or none response triggered when there appears to be no secure route for exploration and no perceived route for escape. It is associated with a suspension of ongoing activity and often followed by a longer-lasting inhibition of exploration. This secondary inhibitor of exploration would in the authors' model lead to depression and would be one explanation for the common association of panic with depression. However, depression might precede panic, and in this case the alteration in the threshold to novelty which can complicate depression and its associated separation anxiety would contribute to the predisposition to panic. As has been pointed out above, internal factors such as endocrine disorders and changes in pCO_2 would also alter the sensitivity of the comparator and predispose to panic.

IMPLICATIONS FOR DRUG TREATMENT

If we assume that in panic disorders the sensitivity of the comparators to novelty is increased to a degree where the panic response is too easily triggered, then the best treatment would be to try to restore the sensitivity of these mechanisms to normal, which might be achieved by increasing the input from 5-HT systems and possibly by decreasing the input from central noradrenergic systems.

The best candidate for such an action would be the tricyclic drugs, in particular those acting on 5-HT systems. The role of action on central noradrenergic systems needs further elucidation.

Other drugs such as beta-blockers may have some effect via action on peripheral noradrenergic systems, and benzodiazepines might block the attacks, perhaps by action on the efferent pathway.

Treatment with the tricyclics would also result in an increase in exploratory behaviour, and this in our model would be accompanied by the relief of depression.

Table 11.1 shows some of the drugs which have been used to treat panic and the authors have reviewed these in more detail elsewhere (Walker and Ashcroft 1989). We would agree with Klein's (1964) pioneering judgement that the only drugs which cause true remission of the attacks with a fairly low incidence of recurrence are the older tricyclics.

Other drugs such as the benzodiazepines or the beta-blockers may suppress components of the panic response but appear to have less effect on the overall syndrome or are associated with a high relapse rate on withdrawal. Drugs such as buspirone may be ineffective (Sheehan *et al.* 1990).

TABLE 11.1. *Drugs which have been evaluated in the treatment of panic disorders*

Drug	Recent References
Tricyclic antidepressants	
imipramine	Zitrin *et al.* (1983)
clomipramine	Johnston *et al.* (1988)
Monoamine oxidase inhibitors	
phenelzine	Solyom *et al.* (1981)
Other antidepressants	
zimelidine	Evans *et al.* (1986)
fluoxetine	Gorman *et al.* (1987)
fluvoxamine	Den Boer *et al.* (1987)
tryptophan	Kahn *et al.* (1987)
trazodone	Mavissakalian *et al.* (1987)
Benzodiazepines	
alprazolam	Ballenger *et al.* (1988)
diazepam	Dunner *et al.* (1986)
clonazepam	Pollack *et al.* (1986)
Beta-blockers	
propranolol	Munjack *et al.* (1985)
Other drugs	
buspirone	Napolliello and Domantoy (1988)
clonidine	Liebowitz *et al.* (1981)

In a double-blind comparison of placebo, clomipramine, and behaviour therapy which was carried out in Aberdeen (Waring 1988), both active treatments proved superior to placebo, clomipramine being effective in 80 per cent of patients in doses of 10–30 mg/d. An interesting phenomenon, also observed by others, is that 30 per cent of patients on clomipramine showed an initial marked exacerbation of panic attacks during the first few days of treatment. The authors are not sure why symptoms initially worsen in these patients but it could represent a preliminary potentiation of noradrenergic mechanisms prior to the onset of action on central 5-HT systems. To explore this possibility the authors carried out an open study with fluoxetine which is a selective 5-HT uptake inhibitor (Lyle *et al.* 1991). The indications are that the drug may be effective and, although the authors saw no exacerbation of panic during the first week of treatment, some patients did experience an increase in generalized anxiety. We are now conducting a double-blind trial of clomipramine, fluoxetine, and placebo which should allow direct comparison of the two drugs.

IMPLICATIONS FOR PSYCHOLOGICAL THERAPIES

It follows from the model that psychological interventions could work by influencing a number of different processes. Since anxiety may be related to the perception of environmental threat, cognitive methods could be helpful. Alternatively, because arousal and selective attention affect perception, training in relaxation or distraction procedures might be beneficial. Flight, alarm, and anxiety change both the external environment and the internal state: therefore, graded exposure to evoking environmental stimuli should be helpful in reducing novelty and hence panic.

Turning to the lower part of the model, visceroception might be altered using cognitive methods or exposure to frightening bodily sensations brought about, for example, by experimental hyperventilation or exposure to feared situations. The sensations should be less frightening if separation anxiety is reduced, for example by promoting secure attachment to the therapist — this could be an important factor in the many studies with a high placebo response (e.g. Ballenger *et al.* 1988). Moreover, such attachment should facilitate exploratory behaviour.

Evidence for efficacy of behaviour therapy

But so much for theory. What evidence is there that behavioural approaches do have an impact on panic?

Most of the early literature, as is well known, concentrated on patients who in addition to panic also had marked avoidance. Most of these patients suffered from agoraphobia or social phobia. Many clinical trials were carried out and have been well reviewed by Marks (1987). There is no doubt that encouraging patients to confront the situations which they fear can be very helpful in terms of reducing phobic avoidance, secondary depression, and the frequency of panic attacks. Examples of procedures with these effects include graded exposure, flooding, and programmed practice.

In the last decade, there has been increasing interest in psychological approaches which target panic *per se*, as opposed to panic-related avoidance behaviour. Indeed, at least one study has suggested that, even in patients with marked avoidance behaviour, exposure to the interoceptive cues associated with panic may be more effective in reducing panic than exposure to environmental triggers. Klosko and Barlow (1987) treated 16 patients with panic disorder and 16 patients with panic disorder plus agoraphobia. The patients with panic disorder received systematic exposure to interoceptive cues whereas the agoraphobics received mainly exposure to external cues. Forty per cent of the agoraphobics were panic free at the end of therapy compared with over 80 per cent of the panic disorder patients.

There is now evidence from several controlled trials that psychological methods which target the panic attacks themselves, rather than the avoidance behaviour, can be very effective (Barlow *et al.* 1984). For example, Klosko and Barlow (1990) reported a comparison of alprazolam and behaviour therapy in the treatment of panic disorder. Sixteen patients were treated using alprazolam, 11 received placebo, 15 were put on a waiting-list and a further 15 received what the authors (Kloskow and Barlow) call 'panic control treatment'. Panic control treatment involves training the patient in relaxation and breathing control, cognitive manoeuvres such as decatastrophization, and interoceptive exposure to feared bodily sensations using, for example, experimental hyperventilation. The percentage of clients completing the study who were free of panic attacks following panic control therapy was 87 per cent compared with 50 per cent for alprazolam, 36 per cent for placebo, and 33 per cent for the waiting-list group. Panic control therapy was significantly better than the placebo or waiting-list conditions, whereas alprazolam therapy was not significantly better than the placebo or waiting-list conditions.

Given that neither drug therapy nor behaviour therapy are completely effective for all patients, there is an *a priori* case for combining behavioural and pharmacological methods. Some cognitive therapists have argued that this may be injudicious as dependence on medication may undermine motivation to learn psychological methods of coping and to stay in distressing conditions until fear subsides. Furthermore, they say it may be important prophylactically for patients to attribute treatment to their own efforts rather than to drug therapy. In practice, it is believed that these difficulties are by no means inevitable. Excellent clinical results can be obtained with a combined approach. For example, Telch *et al.* (1985) carried out a small study with 29 patients — imipramine plus exposure, placebo plus exposure, and imipramine with anti-exposure instructions (imipramine was given in a high dose). In this moderately depressed sample, the best results were obtained by combining imipramine and exposure. Mavissakalian *et al.* (1983) reported a trial of imipramine on its own, or combined with programmed practice, with 18 agoraphobic patients. The authors (Mavissakalian *et al.*) concluded that imipramine possesses an antiphobic effect and that this is substantially enhanced with programmed practice. Differences were less marked on panic and anxiety. Waring (1988) also found advantages in combining behaviour therapy and clomipramine: behaviour therapy helped to reduce avoidance behaviour and improved the maintenance of therapeutic gains.

A PRACTICAL APPROACH TO THE MANAGEMENT OF PANIC ATTACKS

Panic occurs in a range of clinical conditions. Patients suffering from primary depression complicated by panic attacks are treated for a depressive illness with full doses of antidepressants or ECT. However, in the presence of panic, it is advisable to start with a small dose of antidepressant, for example 25 mg clomipramine at night, to avoid the precipitation of more severe panic.

Because there is evidence that behavioural and psychopharmacological approaches are effective in the treatment of panic with, or without, phobic avoidance, where resources are available, patients should be given a choice. The therapist should explain the advantages and disadvantages of both. If resources do not permit this, the authors recommend commencing treatment with a small dose of clomipramine (10 mg at night). If panic has not subsided within 4 or 5 days, the dose should be doubled and then, after a further 2–3 days, increased to a maximum daily dose of 30 mg clomipramine. The possibility of an initial upsurge of symptoms is discussed with patients and they are encouraged to persist with the drug with the expectation that improvement will follow. They are seen frequently during the early days of treatment and, as soon as there is improvement in panic, they are encouraged to overcome phobic avoidance.

If patients fail to tolerate clomipramine, fluoxetine, doxepin, or imipramine are then tried. Doxepin and imipramine seem less potent but they are also less likely to precipitate severe panic symptoms. Unfortunately, fluoxetine is only routinely available in a dose of 20 mg: Schneir *et al.* (1990) used a starting dose of 5 mg and suggested that this increased acceptability.

Very occasionally, diazepam 5 mg twice daily is added to the regime to facilitate the introduction of clomipramine, but the diazepam is always withdrawn within a week.

Drug treatment should be maintained for 6 months and follow-up continued for at least 12 months.

Patients who choose behaviour therapy all initially receive training in cue-controlled relaxation (with an audio cassette recording for home practice). This greatly reduces the number of drop-outs and minimizes the distress experienced during *in vivo* or interoceptive exposure. The emphasis of treatment differs depending on symptoms. Patients with significant avoidance are treated using graded self-directed *in vivo* exposure, having first received graded exposure to these situations in imagination during clinic sessions: patients are first relaxed, or hypnotized if they are able and willing, and asked to imagine as vividly as possible a fear-inducing situation. Keeping the image as vivid as possible, they are then encouraged to practise their cue-controlled relaxation and to use previously rehearsed coping statements. Patients whose panic is not situationally cued are exposed using imagery, hypnotic suggestion, or hyperventilation to feared bodily situations. As with phobic patients, they are given practice in ameliorating their distress by means of relaxation and coping statements. For both groups, efforts are directed at modifying anxiety-provoking images and thoughts by providing the patient with basic information about the psychophysiology of anxiety and by using simple cognitive methods such as decatastrophization.

The authors recommend combined drug therapy and behaviour therapy for those patients who either have severe panic or are non-responders.

Waring's (1988) trial of clomipramine with, and without, behaviour therapy was carried out in the early 1980s. These patients are currently being followed up to evaluate the long-term effectiveness of clomipramine therapy, behaviour therapy, and combined drug–behaviour therapy.

CONCLUSIONS

Panic attacks with, or without, avoidance behaviour can be treated effectively using one of several drugs or behavioural methods. The authors have presented a model which they believe sheds some light on how these methods work.

ACKNOWLEDGEMENTS

Figure 11.1 and Table 11.1 are reproduced with permission from Walker and Ashcroft (1989) p. 302 and p. 309.

BIBLIOGRAPHY

Ashcroft, G.W. (1972). Modified amine hypothesis for the aetiology of affective illness. *Lancet*, 573–77.
Ashcroft, G.W. (1973). Affective disorders — clinical aspects. In *Biochemistry and mental illness* (eds L.L. Iversen and S.P.R. Rose). London.
Ashcroft, G.W. Palomo, T., Salzen, E.A., and Waring, H.L. (1987). Anxiety and depression: a psychobiological approach. *Psicopatologia (Madrid)*, **7**, 155–62.

Ballenger, J.C., Burrows, G.D., DuPont, D.L., Lesser, I.M., Noyes, R., Pecknold, J.C. *et al.* (1988). Alprazolam in panic disorder and agoraphobia: results from a multicentre trial — 1. Efficacy in short-term treatment, *Archives of General Psychiatry*, **45**, 413–22.

Barlow, D.H., Cohen, A.S., Waddell, M., Vermilyea, J.A., Klosko, J.S., Blanchard, E.B., and Di Nardo, P.A. (1984). Panic and generalised anxiety disorders: nature and treatment. *Behavior Therapy*, **15**, 431–49.

Den Boer, J.A., Westenberg, H.G.M., Kamerbeek, W.O.J., Verhoevan, W.M.A., and Kahn, R.S. (1987). Effect of serotonin uptake inhibitors in anxiety disorders. A double-blind comparison of clomipramine and fluvoxamine. *International Journal of Clinical Psychopharmacology*, **2**, 21–32.

Costall, B., Domeney, A.M., and Naylor, R.J. (1982) Behavioural and biochemical consequences of persistent over stimulation of mesolimbic dopamine systems in the rat. *Neuropharmacology*, **21**, 327–35.

Dunner, D.L., Ishiki, D., Avery, D.H., Wilson, L.G., and Hyde, T.S. (1986). Effect of alprazolam and diazepam on anxiety and panic attacks in panic disorder: a controlled study. *Journal of Clinical Psychiatry*, **47**, 458–60.

Ellison, G., Handel, J., Rogers, R. *et al.* (1975). Tricyclic antidepressants: effects on extinction and fear learning. *Pharmacology Biochemical Behaviour*, **3**, 7–11.

Evans, L., Kenardy, J., Schneider, P., and Hoey, H. (1986). Effect of a selective serotonin uptake inhibitor in agoraphobia with panic attacks. A double-blind comparison of zimelidine, imipramine and placebo. *Acta Psychiatrica Scandinavica*, **73**, 49–53.

Gorman, J.M., Liebowitz, M.R., Fyer, A.J., Goetz, D., Campeas, R.B., Fyer, M.R. (1987). An open trial of fluoxetine, *Journal of Clinical Psychopharmacology*, **7**, 329–32.

Gray, J.A. (1982). In *The neuropsychology of anxiety: an inquiry into the functions of the septo-hippocampal system*. Oxford University Press, New York.

Johnston, D.F., Troyer, I.E., and Whitsett, S.F. (1988). Clomipramine treatment of agoraphobic women. *Archives of General Psychiatry*, **45**, 453–9.

Kahn, R.S., Herman, G.M., Westenberg, M., Verhoeven, W.M.A., Gispen-de-Wied, C.C., and Hamerbeek, W.O.T. (1987). Effect of a serotonin precursor and uptake inhibitor in anxiety disorders: a double-blind comparison of 5-hydroxytryptophan, clomipramine and placebo. *International Journal of Clinical Psychopharmacology*, **2**, 33–45.

Klein, D.F. (1964). Delineation of two drug-responsive anxiety syndromes. *Psychopharmacologia*, **5**, 397–403.

Klosko, J. and Barlow, D.H. (1987). Cited in Barlow, D.H. and Cerny, J.A. (1988). *Psychological treatment of panic*. Guilford Press, New York.

Klosko, J. and Barlow, D.H. (1990). A comparison of alprazolam and behavior therapy in the treatment of panic disorder. *Journal of Consulting and Clinical Psychology*, **58**, 77–84.

Liebowitz, M.R., Fyer, A.J., McGrath, P., and Klein, D.F. (1981). Clonidine treatment of panic disorder. *Psychopharmacology Bulletin*, **17**, 122–3.

Lyle, A., Walker, L.G., Logan, E.S. and Ashcroft, G.W. (1992). Fluoxetine in the treatment of panic attacks: an open trial. (In preparation.)

Makanjoula, R.O.A., Hill, C., Maben, I., Dow, R.C., and Ashcroft, G.W. (1977*a*).

An automated method for studying explanatory and stereotyped behaviour in rats. *Psychopharmacology*, **52**, 271–7.

Makanjuola, R.O.A., Hill, G., Dow, R.C., Campbell, G., and Ashcroft, G.W. (1977*b*). The effect of psychotropic drugs on exploratory and stereotypical behaviour of rats studied in a 'holeboard'. *Psychopharmacology*, **55**, 67–74.

Makanjuola, R.O.A., Dow, R.C., and Ashcroft, G.W. (1980). Behavioural responses to stereotactic controlled injections of monoamine neurotransmitters into the accumbens and caudateputation nuclei. *Psychopharmacology*, **7**, 227–31.

Makanjuola, R.O.A., Salzen, E.A., and Ashcroft, G.W. (1992). The role of the ventral pallidum and the mediation of exploratory behaviour in the rat. (In preparation.)

Marks, I.M. (1987). *Fears, phobias and rituals*. Oxford University Press, New York.

Mason, S.T. and Fibiger, H.C. (1979). Noradrenaline and selective attention. *Life Science*, **25**, 1949–56.

Mavissakalian, M., Michelson, L., and Dealy, R.S. (1983). Pharmacological treatment of agoraphobia: imipramine versus imipramine with programmed practice. *British Journal of Psychiatry*, **143**, 348–55.

Mavissikalian, M., Perel, J., Bowler, K., and Dealy, R. (1987). Trazodone in the treatment of panic disorder and agoraphobia with panic attacks. *Journal of Clinical Psychiatry*, **144**, 785–7.

Munjack, D.J., Rebal, R., Shaner, R., Staples, F., Braun, R., and Leonard, M. (1985). Imipramine versus propranolol for the treatment of panic attacks: a pilot study. *Comprehensive Psychiatry*, **26**, 80–9.

Napolliello, M.J. and Domantoy, A.G. (1988). Newer Clinical studies with buspirone. In *Buspirone: a new introduction to the treatment of anxiety* (ed. M. Lader). Royal Society of Medicine, London.

Pollack, M.N., Tesar, G.E., and Rosenbaum, J.F. (1986). Clonazepam in the treatment of panic disorder and agoraphobia: a one-year follow-up. *Journal of Clinical Psychopharmacology*, **6**, 302–4.

Schneir, F.R., Liebowitz, M.R., Davies, S.O., Fairbanks, J., Hollander, E., Campeas, R., and Klein, D.F. (1990). Fluoxetine in panic disorder. *Journal of Clinical Psychopharmacology*, **10**, 119–21.

Sheehan, D.V., Raj, A.B., Sheehan, K.H., and Soto, S. (1990). Is buspirone effective for panic disorder? *Journal of Clinical Psychopharmacology*, **10**, 3–11.

Solyom, L., Heseltine, G.F.D., McClure, D.J., Solyom, C., Ledwedge, B., and Steinberg, G. (1973). Behaviour therapy versus drug therapy in the treatment of phobic neurosis. *Canadian Psychiatric Association Journal*, **18**, 25–32.

Solyom, C., Solyom, L., LaPierre, Y., Pecknold, J., and Morton, L. (1981). Phenetzine and exposure in the treatment of phobias. *Biological Psychiatry*, **16**, 239–47.

Telch, M.J., Agras, W.S., Taylor, C.B., Roth, W.T., and Gallen, C.C. (1985). Combined pharmacological and behavioral treatment for agoraphobia. *Behaviour Research and Therapy*, **23**, 325–35.

Walker, L.G. and Ashcroft, G.W. (1989) Pharmacological approaches to the treatment of panic. In *Panic disorder: theory, research and therapy* (ed. R. Baker). Chichester.

Waring, H.L. (1988). An investigation into the nature and response to treatment of panic attacks in general practice attenders. MD Thesis. University of Aberdeen.

Zitrin, C.M., Klein, D.F., Woerner, M.G., and Ross, D.C. (1983). Treatment of phobias — 1. Comparison of imipramine, hydrochloride and placebo. *Archives of General Psychiatry*, **40**, 125–38.

Index

DATE DUE

APR 1 9 2001			
MAR 1 8 2002			
OCT 2 8 2002			

Demco, Inc. 38-293